YOUR EMOTIONS AND YOU: A WORKBOOK

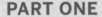

PART ONE

Emotions 101

This part of the book will provide you
with a deeper understanding of emotions:
what they are and how they impact us in
all of life's arenas. You'll also learn some
general tools for managing them.
Get ready for Emotions 101!

CHAPTER ONE

An Introduction to Emotions

This chapter starts off with an overview of emotions, what impacts your emotions, and how your emotions impact you. You'll see that emotions are involved in everything, you'll learn what emotional regulation consists of, and finally, you'll take a quiz to see how well you currently regulate your emotions.

The Undeniable Power of Emotions

We experience myriad emotions daily, but we seldom consider: What is an emotion, anyway? The words *emotion*, *feeling*, and *mood* are used interchangeably, but they are actually quite different. Researchers continue to propose new theories of how they all function. For now, let's strip them down to the basics.

Emotions: An emotion is a complex pattern of reactions—a biochemical message issued by your brain, logging its perceptions about what's happening within and around you. The stimulus that spurs an emotion can be internal, like a thought or memory. Or it can be external: seeing, hearing, smelling, or sensing something familiar and comforting—or unexpected and alarming. These neurochemical messages are experienced as emotions.

Why do we need them? They can help us maneuver through our lives, helping us determine how to respond to specific situations. They can inspire good choices or, perhaps, not-so-good choices. They can even save our lives. Here are a few examples:

- Fear can help us steer away from danger.

- Anger can ignite the fighting spirit to protect our safety or rights. It can inspire us to stand up for the rights of others, too.

- Love can help us choose who to get close to, not to mention helping us snag a date for Saturday night.

Feelings: A feeling is the result of such emotions. Feelings are called feelings, well, because we *feel* them. They are similar to the physical states the body experiences, such as hunger or pain. Body sensations are components of feelings. Think about what happens to your body when you feel fear: Are your muscles tightened? Is your jaw clenched? Are you fighting to catch your breath? Are the hairs on your arms standing at attention? That's physical evidence of fear.

Feelings may also involve interpretations, judgments, or assumptions about what's going on around us, shaped by experience or something we've learned. For example, you might see a dog and experience fear. Your assumption—*Wait, I was once chased by a snarling dog just like that one!*—would be that the animal could harm you. If I see a dog, I might have a very different response. I might experience excitement or an increase in energy. My interpretation—*I grew up with pups! I love them!*—is that I'd love to give that pooch a scratch behind the ears and get that tail wagging!

Moods: A mood can involve both emotions and feelings, but it is longer lasting. Emotions are our initial, immediate reactions to events. Most last just a few moments, and some mere seconds. It's how we interpret, respond to, and fuel emotions that keep them hanging around, extending into a mood. Here's one way to think of it: A mood is a more persistent state of feeling. It has come to stay for a while.

Our emotions influence how we view and respond to our world. They can be useful and life affirming; they can even help drive us to achieve our goals. They can also be disruptive, distracting, and even painful. Nonetheless, they're an essential part of what we've experienced and who we are. The power of emotions in influencing our physical health, our mental state, our relationships, and our general well-being cannot be denied. Understanding them can *feel* so empowering.

How Our Emotions Impact Us

Now that you have a better understanding of what an emotion is, let's talk about how they influence us. Every day, all day, signals for emotions are firing off in our brains like fireworks, impacting us in both positive and negative ways. The impact can be obvious, such as getting so enraged at the boss that we shout, "I quit!" It can be more subtle, too, like the contentment that arises from sipping a cup of herbal tea.

From birth, emotions provide powerful information to secure our safety. They tell us who cares for us and who doesn't, whom to love and whom to be wary of. Emotions help us decide how and when to react. They can shape our health, mental and physical. Emotions help us make vital decisions and they can tell us when to make changes. They can also motivate us to attain the goals we've set to achieve genuine change. Let's take a closer look.

Emotions Send Us Important Signals

For the most part, our brains are pretty, well, primitive. Don't take that statement personally, dear brain. It's just biology. Routinely, our prefrontal cortex (PFC) is in charge of our executive functions, our "higher order" thinking. But when serious threats confront us, an older, more primitive part of our brain takes over.

When our safety becomes critical, the oldest part of our brain, the limbic system, goes into action. It tells the PFC, "Step aside, chum. I'm in charge now!" It swiftly scans for threats and signals us to fight, flee, or freeze. Its message: We can slug our way to safety, run like hell, or just play dead.

Ever get a vague sense of unease when walking to your car in an unfamiliar neighborhood? That's your limbic system telling you to watch for danger. Ever get irritated at a colleague who takes credit for your idea? That's your limbic system alerting you to a threat to your livelihood.

But not every situation calls for fight, flight, or freeze. Our limbic system often hijacks our emotions in everyday life, leaving us feeling anger or anxiety that is totally out of proportion to the situation at hand. Yikes! That's why learning to regulate emotions is so important. When something triggers strong emotions, knowing how to manage them keeps us from having to respond to every situation like it's life or death.

Emotions Affect Our Capacity to Make Decisions

Making decisions can call for a recipe of reason and emotion, and the big decisions can require the most ingredients. For example, on paper, many colleges can meet our needs. Does Home-spun University "feel" like the right school to attend? Or is Momentous Tech a better choice? Who has the strongest curriculum? Where do I want to live for four years? Which is most affordable? Whose programs can land me an ideal job? We've weighed the pros and cons, but what helps us make the final pick? Inevitably, it's the feeling in our gut. This is when emotions can actually be helpful.

But, sometimes, when we experience a strong emotion, we can get sucked into tunnel vision. We lose our PFC, the limbic system takes over, and emotion takes charge. We stop seeing options and focus instead on a limited number of factors, maybe even just one. Let's say I feel fear when stepping onto an elevator. That causes me to avoid them. I see only a choice between plummeting to an uncertain fate and surviving to take the stairs instead. That's fine . . . until the interview for my dream job is on the 66th floor! Choices like these are when emotional-regulation skills become vital. You'll find lots of those in upcoming chapters.

Emotions Motivate Us

Emotions motivate us to take action to increase positive emotions and minimize the probability of feeling negative ones.

What motivates us? We are motivated to seek food, water, and shelter and, in some cases, to procreate. Well, those are the baseline needs, anyway. At the base level, emotions increase the probability of survival and keeping the family line alive. But we need more, of course. Our behaviors are also influenced by a desire for social approval and acceptance. We are driven to build social bonds, to form and maintain human relationships and teams. We look to affiliate, to belong to something. We desire harmony, closeness, and love. Here are some examples of how emotions help us achieve this:

- Emotions signal to us that something is right or wrong.

- Anger can motivate us to stand up for ourselves or others.

- Guilt drives us to make amends for ways we may have hurt others.

- Shame motivates us to refrain from behaviors that could result in rejection from our community.

- Fear helps us elude dangerous situations.

- Satisfaction can be the inner reward for "getting it right."

These all help us thrive in a community, whether we've chosen to join it, were born into it, or were invited in by others.

Emotions Spur Us toward Reaching Goals

Beyond the motivation to seek food, water, and affiliation, more challenging goals consistently crop up during our lives. Powerful emotions can motivate us to achieve difficult things. The emotions that trigger this process aren't necessarily always positive, but they can provoke positive changes. For example:

- Love can motivate us to risk our own safety to keep our loved ones safe from harm.

- Anger and disgust about injustice can arouse activism.

- Envy can embolden us to work hard and acquire items or status that other people have acquired, potentially creating a more comfortable life for ourselves and our families.

Olympic athletes, for example, can be powered by an emotional "energy drink" comprised of the following:

- Pride, desiring to be the very best in their sport.

- Love for country, aiming to make their patriotic peers back home proud.

- Envy of past athletes, igniting the desire to break their records.

Great passion drives us to continue when success seems improbable, even impossible. It causes us to feel fear, but can also inspire the courage to continue. Emotion can be the driving force that galvanizes us to take action, to take strides toward change. So harnessing it can be integral in our lives.

Emotions Affect How We Think About and React to Events

Our moods can influence our interpretations of routine, everyday occurrences as well as more important events.

When we feel anxious or afraid, we may interpret cues that would normally be perceived as nonthreatening or neutral as deeply frightening. Remember the last time you went to a scary movie? When you got home, a knife-wielding maniac seemed to be lurking in every shadow, right? The movie did its job, and so did your emotions, though maybe a little too well.

When we are sad, it can shape our responses. Someone rejected our invitation to coffee? That can feel like a precursor of a grim life of loneliness and despair. When we're in a happy or neutral mood, we can brush it off and go to the Starbucks drive-through window instead.

The lesson: If we allow our emotions to drive our behavior and actions at all times, that can result in significant problems. For example, I want to share some positive news, but my pal Amy doesn't return my text. She's ghosting me, right? My response: Blow up her phone with angry accusations. She deserves it! Later, I learn that she was in an important work meeting and couldn't answer her phone. As you can see, regulating our emotions helps us keep our relationships intact. And losing control of them . . . sorry, Amy.

Emotions Hold Sway over Our Relationships

From the time we are born, we are dependent on others for physical survival and psychological well-being. There's no way around that. A remarkable number of emotions occur during interactions with those folks we count on. Emotions help us express ourselves when we cannot find words; they communicate to our loved ones what we need. Fear, anger, shame, guilt, love, and joy are ways people come to know what is important to us.

Emotions in families can spur chain reactions of responses, both negative and positive. Negative reactions can circle back endlessly, creating conflict and emotional pitfalls as they go. When it comes to our significant others, whether or not they know it, they provide us with the stimuli for the emotions we express. They're also on the receiving end of the emotions they've triggered.

Studies show that we are more likely to be depressed if we are part of a "distressed couple" rather than in a serene relationship. Couples who experience consistent conflict in their relationship are more likely to fall victim to substance abuse, anxiety disorders, and health woes. Finding peace in our relationships, meanwhile, typically improves our health and sense of well-being. In a study of military spouses, the routine expression of positive emotions between partners increased resiliency to stress and depression.

Emotions Impact Our Physical Health

Managing our emotions can achieve more than making us feel better mentally. There is solid medical evidence that indicates feeling happier can make us feel better physically. And feeling bad mentally can lead to, literally, feeling bad all over.

Studies clearly indicate that negative emotions such as anger and anxiety are implicated in a panorama of health issues, including heart disease, cancer, arthritis, diabetes, and even the common cold. Experts have linked depression, anger, and anxiety to cardiovascular disease. Physical symptoms such as lethargy, weakness, severe headaches, and abdominal discomfort often turn out to be mental health concerns in disguise, researchers say.

Don't get too alarmed, though. Feeling better emotionally can lead to feeling better physically. Studies indicate that positive emotions such as joy, gratitude, and contentment can be indicators of superior health. Positive emotions such as love, contentment, and happiness have been linked to improved immune-system function, less severe levels of pain, and lower death rates among people with chronic disease. Research suggests that optimism may even protect against pulmonary disease.

The bottom line: Learning to respond to the emotions we feel as a part of everyday life in a more flexible and resilient way can help us live longer, healthier lives.

What Impacts Our Emotions?

In the same way that emotions shape our sense of wellbeing each day, external and internal factors can also shape our emotions. Both big and small developments can inspire emotions we simply don't see coming. Events in our environment, from simple interactions with people to significant life transitions, all affect how we feel. Even the weather can inspire emotions. Imagine the joy a beautiful spring day can bring. And remember the melancholy brought on by that last rainy afternoon—especially on the weekend!

Other factors can also set off emotions. What we eat can fuel our sense of well-being. Did you have a good night's sleep or did you toss and turn? Big test tomorrow? Meeting with the boss? Our thoughts and assumptions about the world can inspire emotions, too. Memories, reflections, speculation, and anticipation can all trigger emotions. Being aware of this can empower us to anticipate and manage such feelings.

Let's look at these external and internal factors a little more closely.

The Environment We're In

During the COVID-19 pandemic, many of us got a firsthand education in how our environment can impact our emotions. The coronavirus crisis sparked an unprecedented torrent of emotions. Many of us knew someone who got very sick or died. None of us were prepared for this. We all coped differently. For example:

- The number of home-renovation projects soared as folks tried to deal with fear, grief, and isolation by improving their immediate environment.

- Cozy loungewear sales experienced unprecedented growth as people sought to soothe themselves.

- The food-delivery business exploded as anxiety-ridden people summoned comfort food to their doorsteps.

Mind you, the nation's angst was already at peak levels after a highly contentious election. Political polarization hit record levels. We could not reach consensus on how to cope with COVID-19, further deepening our divisions. Then, at the peak of the pandemic, the killing of George Floyd by a Minnesota police officer sparked an unprecedented wave of social unrest. Protesters flooded the nation's streets, expressing their outrage over police killings of people of color.

Add to all that an array of wildfires, hurricanes, economic upheaval, celebrity deaths, and canceled sports and entertainment events—all fueling deep-seated uncertainty. Like it or not, it was a lesson in how emotions, moods, and the actions of people in our environment impact us.

Even during "normal" times, without all of the upheaval of the years 2020 and 2021, we are constantly faced with stimuli that impact our emotions. In our home, workplace, school, and community, we receive messages from our environment that set off emotional responses. Emotions can be contagious, passed from person to person. Humans automatically mimic the facial expressions, voice tone, and body language of others—even if they pick them up via a Zoom call or FaceTime session.

No matter our circumstances, managing our emotions can help us cope more effectively with challenging situations. We've made it this far, right? And, with some more tools, we can make it even farther!

Our Thoughts

How we think influences our emotions. Let's go back to middle school for a moment. Imagine being in the cafeteria. You've grabbed your tray and piled it with food. You're walking toward a table filled with new friends. As you get nearer, you can hear them laughing. What is your immediate reaction? If you decide they are laughing at you, you may feel angry, stomp away, and never speak to them again. If you interpret their laughter as a response to something funny, you will feel excited to join the fun.

How we think influences how we feel and how we behave. How I feel and behave may be very different from how you feel and behave in the very same situation. While thoughts can trigger emotions, they can also help us assess whether these thoughts are realistic and assist us in making changes. This is at the core of cognitive behavioral therapy and is well represented in the exercises in this book.

Our Previous Experiences

If we had a certain emotion in a previous situation, we are more likely to have that emotion in future situations that seem similar. We often react in the present moment to old scenarios if we are unmindful of being in the present. We can have obsolete emotional responses that can cause us to react irrationally and in an emotionally dysregulated manner.

Our emotional mind can also react to situations in the present based on past experiences even when the current conditions are very different. Ever notice yourself playing out old relationships in current relationships? That is this concept in action. Ever feel like you married one of your parents? That's also this concept in action.

Past trauma has a strong impact on our emotions. Trauma can cause survivors to feel emotions very strongly when faced with reminders of the traumatic event. It can also cause people to numb out or dissociate to avoid trauma triggers. If past trauma affects your life, know that there is help available. A therapist can help you learn to cope and eventually thrive. There are some useful resources on page 143 that may also help inform you about the role of trauma in our lives.

Reinforcement

All animals, including human beings, are influenced by the consequences of their behaviors. In behavioral terms, this is called reinforcement. All day, every day, we are being reinforced for our behaviors and reinforcing others' behaviors through our reactions.

If we display an emotion that causes people to respond in ways that are beneficial to us, we are more likely to display that emotion again in similar situations. For example, if I become angry at a salesclerk and get a refund or better service because of it, I am more likely to become a serial complainer in stores. If I show sadness and cry when someone is angry at me, and that person stops yelling and comforts me, I am more likely to cry in the future when someone is angry with me. This is the behavioral principle of reinforcement in action.

If I experience something positive or the removal of something negative when displaying a specific behavior, I am more likely to engage in that behavior.

Life Changes

Big shifts in our lives can greatly impact our emotions. They can be hurtful, disruptive events like divorce, losing a job, or the death of a loved one. Happy events can impact us emotionally, too. Though they are wonderful developments, falling in love, the birth of a child, or landing a great new job can create stress, too.

Significant changes and transitions to new stages in life can shape our emotions as we adjust to the big changes. For some people, such change can be exciting. But, for many others, these moments can be frightening, unnerving, and even overwhelming.

Remember how primitive I told you our brains are? Well, when impactful moments arrive in our lives, our brain sometimes can't cope with them. Interestingly, our brains can interpret any life change as a threat. They're just looking out for us, after all. They can't be sure if the change is positive or not; They only have past experiences to go on.

While our brain catches up, we can experience an increase in stress. We may feel fear and perhaps even grief. Even if the change is good, we can experience a sense of loss, instinctively longing for the ways things were before. Not surprisingly, we can also get tangled up in confusion as we adjust to a new reality. Change can be good, but it's seldom easy.

Sleep

Ever wake up on wrong side of the bed? It's something most of us have experienced. How much sleep we get can impact our emotions. Current research indicates that there is a bidirectional relationship between mental health and sleep. It can be a vicious cycle; insomnia and other sleep disorders impact our emotional state, and, in turn, our emotional state impacts our sleep.

Improving sleep can have a big impact on our emotional reactivity. Even brain activity during sleep profoundly affects our emotional health. Getting enough REM sleep helps our brains process emotional information effectively, since that's when we generally dream. A lack of sleep can be especially harmful to our efforts to process positive emotional content.

Having consistent problems getting to sleep? Get some help. Diagnosing and treating sleep issues such as obstructive sleep apnea can have a profoundly positive effect on your mental health. Improving "sleep hygiene" can also be highly effective. This can include:

- Developing a consistent sleep schedule.

- Avoiding caffeine and alcohol for at least four hours before bed.

- Using your bed only for sleep and sex.

- Cutting off use of all electronics 30 minutes before bed.

   Remember: Sleep matters.

Emotions and Prejudice

Prejudice—a "preconceived opinion"—can be manifested in a negative attitude toward a person or group. Unlike some of the emotions we've talked about in this book, it's not based on actual experience. It occurs *before* someone has had an actual interaction with a person or group.

Prejudice can invoke emotional responses, ranging from mild nervousness to extreme hatred. Prejudice can spur thought-provoked actions, too, including harsh judgments and assumptions. Behavioral actions can include discrimination and even violence.

We've talked about how emotion encourages us to include people in our lives. For example:

- Love causes us to want to be closer.

- Happiness inspires us to share common positive experiences.

- Sadness causes us seek soothing and support.

But prejudice can drive us to exclude people. "Social distancing"—not the "six feet apart" kind we experienced during the pandemic—spurs individuals and groups to differentiate themselves from one another. It can be as simple as folks who cheer for different sports teams or who have attended schools they're proud of. But it can also empower them to compete for social status. The tools people apply during this process can be toxic. For example:

- Anger can drive us to want to control others.

- Contempt makes us want to force other people to change.

- Fear makes us cling to the concept that our group—its history, beliefs, practices—is superior.

When we feel threatened, we often tamp down fear with hatred. That other group is fundamentally bad, we tell ourselves. This can serve an affiliative function by drawing the "in group" together, but it also fuels prejudices and bias. That can feed further social distancing.

These biases can even become implicit. We come to accept these feelings as actual truth, rather than as just a theory, a belief, or a fear instilled in us by others. The political polarization that grips our nation is evidence of this; it can be more important to some folks to win an argument than it is to be accurate, thoughtful, or kind. The risk: We grow bitter, we demonize those we disagree with, and, in the end, we are unable to compromise on anything.

It can be tough to terminate this cycle. Sure, the world is full of such prejudice. What can one person do? Regulating our emotions stokes our "emotional intelligence" (we'll explore this concept more on page 14), allowing us to recognize implicit bias before it gets stuck in our psyche. Increased contact with people from different groups, with varied backgrounds, can increase positive emotions, decrease negative emotions, and deflate fear, hatred, and prejudice.

Gaining such maturity is an investment in our own mental health, but it's also good for the whole planet. It empowers us to see and appreciate our shared humanity.

Nutrition

Food does impact mood! The growing field of nutritional psychiatry is finding many correlations between what we eat and our day-to-day emotions. What's more, excessive dieting can impact your emotional state, increasing your vulnerability to negative emotions. So can eating too much or indulging in too many rich foods.

Recent studies compared the following diets with regard to rates of depression:

- A traditional Mediterranean diet, mostly consisting of vegetables, fruits, nuts, seeds, fish, legumes, and whole grains.

- A traditional Japanese diet, mostly consisting of fish, tofu, natto, seaweed, steamed rice, noodles, and fresh or pickled fruits and vegetables.

- A typical "Western" diet, mostly consisting of processed foods, which are frequently high in fat and sugar. (That's what many of us eat in the United States.)

Researchers concluded that the risk of depression was 25 to 35 percent lower in those who ate the traditional diets. Research also indicates that folks seem to experience higher levels of hunger when angry or joyful. Experiencing fear or sadness can propel your appetite, too. Of all those emotions, impulsive eating was rated most common when people are angry. It's clear that managing what we eat can help us manage how we feel.

What Is Emotional Regulation?

We can't just switch our emotions on and off, but we can get better at regulating them. In short, emotional regulation is defined as the ability to influence your emotions. The process involves strategies such as identifying emotions and rethinking challenging situations. It can also involve being more accepting of both positive and negative emotional experiences. Sometimes when we start to feel negatively, we might feel upset about feeling upset, which can amplify the emotion. Acceptance involves looking at your feelings and letting them play out without judgment.

You can think of emotional regulation as a coping strategy for whenever you experience an intense, disruptive emotion—a feeling that's just "too much." The ability to monitor and manage our emotions can result in stronger relationships, greater success in the workplace, and improved long-term health. It can also make us feel better *right now*.

Like it or not, emotions are flawed. They don't offer us the whole picture, and that can trip us up. When we are overly emotional, there is little room for the balanced thought that produces our best thinking and actions. Emotional regulation allows us to *choose* how we respond, to align with our goals and values, rather than simply reacting out of instinct. It may be momentarily satisfying to go off on someone in anger, but it could be hurtful to the long-term goal of maintaining that relationship. It can feel *soooo* good to hit the snooze button and stay in bed, but that hurts the short-term goal of being on time for work.

Emotional Intelligence in the Workplace

When Daniel Goleman's 1995 book *Emotional Intelligence* popularized the concept, business leaders were quick to agree that success on the job is strongly influenced by qualities such as an aptitude for partnering well with workmates and the ability to control our emotional responses.

People with high emotional intelligence are able to accurately identify and label emotions and use emotional information to guide their thinking and behavior. They can adjust their emotions to different environments and know how to handle interpersonal relationships extremely well. This makes for successful workers and effective leaders. Think back to an unpleasant experience you lived through with a salesperson or a customer service rep. Surely they didn't have an ideal outcome in mind, right? Perhaps that worker was lacking in emotional intelligence.

No matter what your job is, training in emotional intelligence results in sharpened performance, better evaluations from management, and improved productivity. Higher levels of emotional intelligence have been linked to greater job satisfaction and reduced burnout rates, especially in folks who work in the public sector.

Can we really measure emotional intelligence? We can, and we are getting better at it. Tests can provide us with information about an individual's self-awareness, self-management aptitude, social awareness skills, and how well they modulate relationships.

A variety of scales, quizzes, and questionnaires have been developed to measure emotional intelligence. Of these, the abilities-based Mayer-Salovey-Caruso Emotional Intelligence Test (MSCEIT) is considered the most accurate and objective by many researchers.

Choosing to use an emotional-regulation technique—especially when an emotion is just too painful to feel—can be healthy indeed. Emotional regulation can be seamless and automatic. But when our approach is effortful and conscious by design (read that as *hard work*) it can be more impactful, especially in the long term. Over time, it gets easier as we master the process and our responses become easier to manage in the moment.

Several factors make regulating emotions difficult. For example:

We are sensitive to emotions and lack the skills to manage them (never fear, that is what this book is for!).

We believe in enduring myths about emotions ("feeling sad makes you weak," etc.).

We get hit with unexpected emotions when we are most vulnerable (hungry, tired, or overwhelmed).

This blueprint for regulating your emotions differs from another concept you may have heard of named *emotional intelligence*. Broadly speaking, emotional intelligence is the ability to understand your emotions, use them to guide your own actions, and to understand the emotions of the people around you.

You can think of emotional regulation as one element of emotional intelligence since it involves being "smarter" about your feelings. Other elements include empathy, motivation, social skills, self-awareness, and self-regulation. This book aims to increase your emotional intelligence by helping you become more aware of your emotions and how to manage them. You will have the opportunity to hone these skills in part 2, where you'll learn to respond to, understand, and harness the power of your emotions.

Key Components of Emotional Regulation

Emotional regulation is made up of many components. Certainly, our ability to adapt, be resilient, and bounce back from emotional experiences is vital. As is our ability to feel empathy and understand the motives of others. Our motivation to regulate our emotions is another factor. Social skills assist us in emotional regulation as they allow us to reduce negative interactions and increase positive interactions with others. Let's take a look at each component.

Self-Awareness

Regulating our emotions requires understanding them. We must be willing to examine how our experiences make us feel. To be self-aware, we learn to respond in ways that are reflective rather than reflexive. Think about that little rubber hammer in the doctor's office. The doc taps your knee, and if your muscles are all wired together properly, your leg kicks out a bit. Reflexes.

Okay, that's fine in the doctor's office. In the real world? Not so much. If we respond to every situation with an instant, reflexive response, be it in the supermarket, in the boss's office, or in the classroom, we might run into some serious problems.

If our lives are at risk, we *do* want to act reflexively and go into fight-or-flight mode. Most days, however, we aren't facing down rabid dogs or Darth Vader. Reflecting on what is happening, and how it makes us feel, is vital to making the best choice that fits with our long-term and short-term goals.

In most situations, and we need to:

1. **Pause.** Take a brief moment to reflect.

2. **Look inward.** Identify the emotion we are feeling.

3. **Assess.** Determine if this emotion is justified by the situation.

4. **Evaluate.** Decide whether it benefits us to immediately act on this emotion.

5. **Act.** Respond accordingly.

   The bottom line: Rewind, and then react reflectively, not reflexively.

Curiosity

Many of us have been socialized to react to various events in a reflexive way. To respond in a reflective, or regulated way, we need to look at situations with curiosity, to respond in ways that are effective for that situation, rather than react to past events or how we have been conditioned to react.

We are conditioned to have automatic, obsolete emotional responses that can get us in trouble. Have you ever assumed that your partner is acting in ways that a previous partner did? Upon reflection, did you need to apologize for your reaction?

Being curious about the current situation and not automatically deciding we know what is happening based on previous experience helps us regulate and decide upon a more effective reaction. And we don't have to create rifts in our relationships and do something we have to apologize for. In these cases, making benign assumptions about the behavior of others is in our own best interests until we have significant evidence to the contrary.

Put simply, curiosity can help us more effectively empathize with the people in our lives. For example, you might be able to piece together clues that someone you know lives in fear of being abandoned. Might that reshape your interactions with them? Adopting a curious mindset about your own emotional responses to people and experiences can be just as empowering.

Self-Compassion

How do you treat a friend who is going through a tough time? With concern, patience, and tenderness, of course. Why don't you treat yourself with the same consideration and caring? We often self-chastise in ways that are brutally critical and judgmental. Kristin Neff, a leading expert in self-compassion who popularized the term, breaks the concept into three elements:

1. **Self-kindness vs. Self-judgment:** Recognizing that humans are imperfect, we should work to soothe ourselves, not focus sharply on our flaws.

2. **Common Humanity vs. Isolation:** Acknowledging that we are not the only ones suffering, we come to terms with the fact that distress and hardship are, like it or not, part of being human.

3. **Mindfulness vs. Overidentification:** Reminding ourselves that thoughts and feelings are simply, well, thoughts and feelings. This prevents us from getting swept away by negative reactivity.

Self-critical thoughts like "You suck!" are perceived by the brain as emotional attacks, which can ignite the fight-or-flight response. That tells our brains to cut loose increased levels of cortisol, a hormone released when we are under stress. High levels of cortisol have been linked with depression, anxiety, and cognitive impairment.

On the other hand, practicing self-compassion sets off the tend-and-befriend response, releasing oxytocin, a hormone connected to love and bonding. A self-compassionate thought might be "I'm doing the best I can." Responding to a difficult situation with a thought like this can increase our sense of calm, making us feel safe. It can also decrease levels of cortisol, easing symptoms of depression and anxiety.

We can better regulate our emotions when we are more aware of the feelings of others. When we attempt to understand, instead of judging or punishing the behaviors and emotions of others, it can inspire us to treat folks very differently. They are not, despite what our reflexive emotions might tell us, just jerks who are trying to hurt us.

Have you ever heard the folktale of Androcles and the Lion? A runaway slave takes shelter in a cave, which turns out to be the den of a lion. A loud, roaring lion. Pretty scary, right? So Androcles thinks to himself, "In this uncharted, urgent, emotional setting, a hungry predator may fail to self-regulate and assess my feelings and motivations. He just may, gulp, eat me!"

But, actually, the lion was neither angry nor famished. He had a thorn jammed painfully in his paw. Androcles removed the barb from the lion's foot, and they subsequently became friends, business partners, and the lead characters in a play by George Bernard Shaw (it's true, look it up).

Let's take the time to assess the angry roars of others. Perhaps they are wounded, too. They may need a hand. This may be a good idea to keep in mind the next time your partner is a bit snappy, your child is a bit sassy, or you come across a grumpy salesclerk. Besides, Hannibal Lecter notwithstanding, they probably won't eat you.

The Benefits of Increased Emotional Regulation

Engaging in emotional regulation can have all these benefits:

- Strengthen our relationships. Responding in a regulated way makes it more likely your partner will respond in understanding and loving ways.

- Empower us to treat those closest to us like we love them, rather than taking out our negative emotions on them.

- Protect us against depression and anxiety.

- Reduce hypersensitivity.

- Help us steer clear of the regrettable situations an emotional reaction can stir up.

- Enable us to live more in accordance with our values.

Failing to regulate our emotions can have these negative effects:

- Undermine our relationships.

- Weaken our performance at work.

- Impede our ability to deal with stress and pressure.

How Well Do I Manage My Emotions?

This self-assessment is intended to measure how well you regulate your emotions. Don't spend a lot of time thinking about your answers; just go with your first gut response. Also, don't try to figure out the "right" answer, the one that you are supposed to give to be well regulated emotionally. Give the most honest answer you can.

Don't worry, this is not your final exam. In fact, there is no final exam. I bet you can manage how you feel about your score, too (if you've been paying attention). Please do not expect a perfect score. Humans are not perfect. Maybe robots are, but robots don't read books about emotional regulation. Ready? Here it goes:

1. I cannot function when I feel upset. .... T **(F)**
2. I treat myself in a compassionate way when I am distressed. .... T **(F)**
3. Others handle their emotions better than I do. .... T **(F)**
4. I can express myself accurately when I feel upset. .... T **(F)**
5. I have no idea how to manage my emotions when I am distressed. ...... T **(F)**
6. I can usually take care of my responsibilities even when I am upset. ... **(T)** F
7. Feelings are not important to me. .... T **(F)**
8. I have nondestructive ways to feel better when I am distressed. .... **(T)** F
9. Emotions cause problems for me. .... **(T)** F
10. I know how I am feeling most of the time. .... T **(F)**
11. I become angry with or ashamed of myself when I feel upset. .... T **(F)**
12. I make good decisions even when I am upset. .... **(T)** F
13. I think I will lose control when I have a strong emotion. .... T **(F)**
14. My feelings are valid and deserve my attention. .... **(T)** F
15. I have no idea how I am feeling much of the time. .... **(T)** F
16. Feeling upset is okay; I can handle it. .... **(T)** F

CONTINUED»

Scoring

Look at the even-numbered statements and total the number of trues: __4__ .
Look at the odd-numbered statements and total the number of falses: __6__ .
Time for math! I'm going to give you 16 points just for answering the questions.
16 + __4__ (even-numbered trues) − __6__ (odd-numbered falses) = __14__ (your score)

0–8: There's work to be done. But that's why you are reading this book, right?

9–16: You're on your way. You can gather more strategies by reading on.

17–24: You've almost got this! Stay focused. It's working!

25–32: You're doing great! There's lots more to learn. Read on!

The Lasting Impact of Emotional Regulation

In the long run, folks who practice emotional regulation cope better with stressors. They are simply more resilient because they have higher levels of tolerance for distress. Emotional regulation can lead to mood improvement and can profoundly affect our choices by creating options we may not have otherwise imagined or considered. In laboratory studies, mastering emotional-regulation strategies is closely linked to well-being and financial success. Being able to regulate emotions leads to the ability to make better decisions within the workplace, leading to financial success. But unchecked emotions can get us in all kinds of trouble.

Emotional dysregulation is a term used in the therapy world that refers to emotional responses that are more intense and last longer than desired (or than indicated by the situation). These over-the-top responses can be hurtful to others and ourselves. They can lead to self-harming behavior, substance abuse, and impulsive, even dangerous, choices.

Emotional dysregulation can interfere with a person's social interactions and relationships at home, in school, or in places where we go to unwind and have fun. Maybe we aren't as skillful at managing our annoyance in our relationships and get a little snappy, or we let our emotions get the best of us and don't meet our school or work deadlines.

The good news is that emotional regulation can be learned. In the next chapter, we'll look more closely at various tools that can help you better manage your emotions.

CHAPTER TWO

Emotional Management Tools

In this chapter, you will be introduced to an array of basic tools that can help you better understand and manage your emotions. These concepts will play a key role in many of the exercises created for you throughout this book, as well as in regulating your emotions in general. Let's take a look!

Building Your Toolkit

Don't you love a good toolkit? With the right collection of tools, all in a tidy little case, you can maintain, repair, and build all sorts of things—including your emotional-regulation skills! The tools in this chapter are grounded in the principles introduced in chapter 1, and all are backed by research.

You won't find any chainsaws or chipper shredders here. Each tool is built on the foundation of being compassionate to yourself and others, and being mindful of the emotions we all experience. They should grow your level of self-awareness. They won't shred anything, except perhaps the tendency to be hypercritical of yourself.

Elements of each of these tools will pop up in this book's exercises from here on out. They should help you understand and manage your emotions, help reduce negativity, and help you harness the power of your emotions to construct the life you truly desire.

It is important to remember that not all of these tools work the same way, or as effectively, for all people. Identify the tools that resonate with you and try them out. You may find that some are more useful than others at certain times. When the subject is you, the expert is . . . wait for it . . . you! Only you can decide what works best for you. Now, get ready to choose your tools.

Journaling

Is something troubling you? Or delighting you? Or frustrating you? Write it down.

Journaling can help you process complex thoughts. It builds your ability to understand your feelings and clears away mental clutter. It stokes self-awareness and curiosity, freeing you from the judgments or assumptions of others. Research indicates that regular journaling can:

- Help ease symptoms of varying health issues.

- Improve cognitive functions.

- Strengthen the immune system.

- Reduce obsessive rumination.

- Shift perspectives, helping us consider multiple possible outcomes of situations.

Imagine, all of that for the cost of a pen and some paper! Here are some ideas to get you started:

- Pick a journaling tool you enjoy. It can be anything from colorful scraps of wrapping paper to a spiral-bound notebook to a handsome leatherbound volume. You can also journal on your laptop or with the notes function on your smartphone.

- Keep your journal private. This keeps your writing free of self-censoring.

- Date your entries. Then you can go back and reflect on the past and see how far you've come.

- Write regularly, every day if you can. That will help you gauge the ebb and flow of your emotions. You may start to identify triggers that set off undesired emotions. But . . .

- Set a finite amount of time to write, whether it be 5 or 15 minutes per day. Free yourself from perfectionism and worrying about punctuation or sentence structure. Just let the thoughts pour out. And when time's up for the day, shut the book.

Mindfulness

Professor Jon Kabat-Zinn, well-known author and founder of the Stress Reduction Clinic at the University of Massachusetts, is widely credited for bringing the concept of mindfulness to the attention of Western cultures. Paraphrasing his operational definition, mindfulness is simply using our awareness to pay attention on purpose in this moment without judgment.

What does this look like in an everyday sense? Say you are doing a brief mindfulness meditation. By slowing down your breathing and simply observing your thoughts, feelings, body, and surroundings—without getting caught up in them—you are able to notice moment-by-moment experiences happening right now, rather than worrying about the future or dwelling in the past.

This makes it easier to choose how you respond to situations instead of reacting in ways that may not help you.

Mindfulness has been found to be effective in:

* Reducing pain and improving physical health.

* Strengthening relationships.

* Boosting distress tolerance and reducing stress.

* Easing symptoms of anxiety and depression.

* Increasing positive feelings.

As simple as it may sound, mindfulness changes how we relate to our world. Mindfulness can make us less reactive, calmer, and just generally happier. It builds self-awareness and curiosity. As therapy, being mindful means being aware and purposefully accepting of your thoughts and emotions.

Before you decide that doing mindful meditation is not for you, consider practicing "everyday" mindfulness while performing daily tasks. While showering, notice the temperature of the water, how it feels against your skin, the smell of the soap, the pressure of the water hitting your body, and so on. It's healthier than spending that time ruminating on your problems while soaking wet. And you need to get clean, anyway! Apply this strategy to ordinary tasks throughout the day, and you will start to see all sorts of positive changes. You'll have a chance to try some mindfulness exercises on pages 74 and 84.

Taking a Nonjudgmental Stance

The mind is made to judge. It's simply decision-making at work. Some things are judged as good; we try to get more of those things. Some things are judged as bad; they earn a "no, thank you." There's nothing inherently wrong with judgments. It's just how the mind works.

Sometimes judgments are helpful. They help keep us safe by steering us away from danger. But when we take judgments as facts, things start to go haywire. We may decide that putting ourselves in certain situations, doing particular activities, or interacting with certain people should be avoided. We may even come to believe that some people *are* either good or bad.

In terms of how we feel about ourselves, taking a nonjudgmental stance allows us to approach and observe our thoughts, urges, and impulses from a compassionate perspective, rather than beating ourselves up over them and feeling guilt and shame.

Nonjudgment isn't about ending all judgments; it is about changing your individual relationship to them. It's essential that we observe judgments as mere thoughts to prevent us getting swept up in their power. Instead of judgements, aim for facts; these are much more helpful in managing the strong emotions that come from judgments.

Let's say you forgot a friend's birthday. If you were judging yourself, you might call yourself a "bad friend." This might lead to all sorts of negative emotions, like shame, that could cause you to avoid your friend because seeing them would cause you to feel bad about yourself. Instead, if you chose to accept the facts of the situation and let go of your judgments of yourself, you could call your friend, wish them a belated happy birthday and take them out for a nice lunch.

Here are some ideas for letting go of judgments:

- Ask yourself, "Is judging effective in this situation?"

- Replace judgments with statements of consequences: "This is helpful because . . . " or "This is harmful because . . . "

- Practice describing people, events, or things in different ways, rather than using words such as *good* or *bad, worthwhile* or *worthless,* and *beautiful* or *ugly.* They are what they are.

- Remember not to judge yourself for judging!

Self-Soothing

Self-soothing is being gentle, kind, comforting, and nurturing to yourself. When some folks hear about self-soothing, they recoil. "I'm not a baby! I'm too old for such things!" Sure, it works on infants. But it can work for grown-ups, too, providing they overcome the feeling they aren't worthy of self-soothing. All humans desire it—dare I say, require it—in order to be mentally healthy. It's particularly helpful when one is going through times of deprivation, like being financially strapped or feeling overwhelmed by caring for the needs of others.

Using the five senses as a launching point, seek out ways to be gentle, nurturing, and kind to yourself. Here are some ideas:

- **Sight:** Sit and watch a sunset or keep a photo of one at your desk or bedside. Paint or draw a picture of someone you care deeply about.

- **Scent:** Immerse yourself in scented candles, essential oils, freshly cut grass, or cookies being baked. Mmmm, cookies . . .

- **Hearing:** Listen to the birds chirping outside, play soothing music, or focus on the sounds of water.

- **Taste:** Brew a cup of tea or coffee, or roll a mint or hard candy around in your mouth.

- **Touch:** Climb into comfy jammies, take a bubble bath, get a massage, or stroke your dog or cat (they will concur that this is a great idea).

And, just for grins, let's add another sense (sort of):

- **Movement:** Enjoy a mindful walk, take a yoga class, or do some simple stretches at home. Experts say you can't oversell the value of stretching.

Cognitive Reappraisal

When we have a strong emotion, it can be hard to see any other perspective than what the emotion is eliciting. Our vision narrows and we tune out all other emotions and thoughts. When we are angry, we tend to focus solely on the emotion of anger and the thoughts that make us angry, and that focus makes us even angrier. This keeps the emotion going far longer than it might otherwise.

Cognitive reappraisal is a way of breaking this cycle. Cognitive reappraisal involves the self-awareness of recognizing that you have fallen into a negative thinking cycle and then changing that cycle to a more effective one. Hopping off this cycle involves changing your thoughts. Taking a moment to look at the situation with curiosity and thinking about what else might be true helps loosen anger's grip on you. It may also elicit more positive emotions.

Let's say you are at the grocery store. Someone in front of you in line not only takes out a bunch of coupons, but also wants to pay with a check and, it turns out, wants their groceries split into several orders. Thoughts like "Arghhh!" or "I am *always* so unlucky!" or "This woman is so inconsiderate!" are going to result in a lot of frustration and other negative emotions for you. But if you start having thoughts like "These things happen" or "Perhaps this woman is down on her luck and needs to portion her money carefully" or "Now I have a chance to read all of the tabloids I would never buy," you can change this frustration to more positive emotions.

Visualization

Take a moment, right here, right now, and make yourself comfortable. Close your eyes. Take a few slow, deep breaths in through your nose and out through your mouth.

Imagine a white light floating above you. Imagine this white light warming and soothing your body, starting at your head and moving down to your shoulders and abdomen, through your arms and legs, and down to your toes and fingertips.

Envision any stress or tension you may feel moving out through your fingers and toes as the white light soothes and softens all areas of your body. Take a few deep breaths, and then open your eyes.

Yay! You just engaged in a stress-reducing visualization. Visualization involves using mental imagery to relax and achieve a calmer state of mind. You can also visualize a peaceful setting or a favorite place, imagining all the sights, sounds, smells, and tactile experiences of that environment.

Visualization helps people ground and center themselves so that they can relate more flexibly to their emotions. In your emotion-regulation toolkit, this is perhaps your most portable tool. After all, you can take your imagination anywhere.

Setting Goals

Ready to set some goals? What? Won't that only add *more* stress to your life?! Hear me out. Setting, working toward, and achieving goals can give us a sense of competence and mastery and make us feel good about ourselves. In turn, this positive self-regard leads to increased confidence.

Setting goals helps stimulate positive emotions such as pride and happiness, especially as they are accomplished. Knocking off a short-term goal can feel like a home run. Attaining a long-range ambition? A grand slam.

It is important to set goals that are difficult enough to be challenging but not impossible to achieve. Rewarding and celebrating small steps toward the goals will help make these aspirations more achievable.

Remember to set both short-term and long-term goals. If you focus only on long-term targets, you can get overwhelmed and feel stuck. For longer-range plans, map them out on a timeline. Along the way, checking off small action steps on a to-do list can set off little bursts of self-satisfaction. For example, if you are working toward a college degree, as you accomplish each assignment and each class, see these achievements as steps toward your final goal.

Acceptance

Inevitably, life involves pain. Pain + nonacceptance = suffering. When we attempt to avoid unpleasant thoughts and feelings, we can actually increase their duration and frequency. They are like little imps that ride around on our shoulders, yammering in our ears. Suppressing negative thoughts and emotions only makes that self-destructive chatter louder.

Steven Hayes, the codeveloper of acceptance and commitment therapy (ACT), promotes acceptance as an alternative to that incessant cycle of scrambling to elude overwhelming emotions. Hayes views acceptance as the active choice to allow unpleasant experiences to exist without trying to deny or alter them. But it is not just acceptance that is key here. It is committing to accepting that the unpleasant experience exists *and* still living the life we aspire to—not waiting until the unpleasant experience goes away before we can truly live.

Unpleasant emotions and experiences are an inevitable—even essential—part of being human. And we can build a sense of competence and mastery when we do not strive to avoid what we fear. Mind you, acceptance does not mean lying down and saying, "Whatever, bring on the pain." It's a process.

Before we attempt to change a situation, we must accurately recognize what the situation is. This requires acceptance. By refusing to back away from seemingly unbearable emotions, we can take steps toward healing—and move through feelings of worry and sadness at the same time.

Validation

Have you ever had the experience of being fire-breathing, nail-spitting angry about something? Did you end up talking to someone who "got it," someone who truly understood why you felt that way? After speaking to that person, were you less upset? That's validation in action.

Validation is listening to and learning about another person's emotions, thoughts, beliefs, and experiences in a nonjudgmental way. Validation strengthens relationships and shows the other person that they are important to you.

When others ignore, reject, or judge our experiences, it can send the message that our emotions are wrong, off-kilter, or weird. This is called invalidation and can make us feel isolated and unsupported. Sometimes, invalidation is a product of others not understanding, and we can be more effective in helping them understand. Here are some things you can say when you think you are starting to be invalidated:

- "I don't think I'm being clear. Let me try to say that in a different way."

- "Can you paraphrase what you hear me saying so that I can find out if I'm saying what I mean to say?"

- "I really appreciate you listening, but I think I am not getting my point across. Can I try this again at a different time?"

Recovering from being invalidated by someone can involve self-validation, which takes self-reflection. You must make it clear to yourself that, even if no one else understands, your experience is valid, makes sense, and is worthy of self-assessment.

Gratitude

Just as acceptance of negative events can be key to attaining good mental health, gratitude for positive events can be just as beneficial. Studies indicate that gratitude leads to higher levels of perceived social support and lower levels of stress and depression. That's because we when we practice gratitude, we see all the awesome things we miss when we don't practice gratitude. So, we notice the cool people in our lives, thank them more often, and feel less stress.

Cultivating gratitude not only makes you feel better, but it can also make you a better person. So, how can you cultivate and practice gratitude? Commit to making a list, daily or weekly, of all the things you are grateful for.

Just like self-soothing, a great way to practice gratitude on the fly is using the senses as a prompt:

- **Sight:** Name one thing you can see that you are grateful for. How about the flowers the neighbor planted?

- **Hearing:** One thing you can hear that you are grateful for. Maybe some David Bowie?

- **Smell:** One thing you smell that you are grateful for. Have we mentioned the scent of baking cookies lately?

- **Touch:** One thing you can touch that you are grateful for. And it doesn't have to be fingers—how about the feeling of standing barefoot in the surf?

- **Taste:** One thing you can taste that you are grateful for. Yum!

Challenge yourself to come up with different things each time you do this exercise.

Making the Most of These Tools

These tools, along with the concepts introduced in part 1, provide the foundation for the exercises you will undertake in chapters ahead. These tools are helpful to practice on their own, too:

- Mindfulness, acceptance, gratitude, validation, and taking a nonjudgmental stance can help you shape your daily mindset.

- Journaling, setting goals, and cognitive reappraisal can all go hand in hand to help you better recognize your emotions and chart desired changes. Even scribbling a note to yourself about your goals for change can count as journaling. Taking a brief moment to confront an unhelpful thought? That's cognitive reappraisal.

- Try incorporating self-soothing and visualization into your winding-down-for-the-day routine.

If you use any of these tools, individually or linked in tandem, you are paving your path to increased understanding and emotional regulation. Throughout part 2, you'll have the chance to put all these tools into action with easy-to-follow exercises that incorporate the concepts discussed so far.

PART TWO

Working with Your Emotions

You've learned a lot about emotions and how they work. Now it's time to wrap your brain around *your* emotions. Chapters 3 through 5 will help you identify your emotions and what triggers them. You'll also get some help managing them, particularly the negative ones. In chapter 6, you'll build upon what you've learned and start harnessing your emotions, synchronizing them to help spur personal growth.

CHAPTER THREE

Understanding Your Emotions

Before you can truly manage your emotions, you must first understand them. The goal is to recognize and accept emotions as they arise and trace them back to their origins. This can be trickier than it sounds. Emotions are complex behavioral responses. Emotions such as anger can actually be other emotions in disguise, like anxiety, hurt, and sadness.

Your current assumptions about your emotions can get in the way of really understanding them. You may need to shed some long-held beliefs about why you feel the way you do before you can change how you relate to them.

Boost Your Self-Awareness

If you aren't aware of your thoughts and feelings, how can you tell what's really going on inside? Self-awareness is vital to understanding what makes us tick. Identifying our preconceived beliefs about emotions is often a first step to self-awareness.

Over the course of our lives, we come to accept various myths about emotions. We learn these from our families, our cultures, and even the media. These myths can get in the way of effectively identifying and expressing emotions in a healthy way. Our state of mind can help perpetuate such myths. In this section, you will learn about the three states of mind and how they impact our success at managing emotions.

Being in a balanced state of mind helps you make decisions linked to your short-term goals, your long-term goals, and your enduring values. Being in the state of Wise Mind means you can balance your emotions and logic. This can help you feel more confident in your decisions and your ability to regulate your emotions. You can believe that you are capable of dealing with difficult situations because *you* are steering the ship, not your emotions. This is the ultimate in emotional regulation! We will return to the concept of Wise Mind throughout the exercises.

What Do You Believe?

In our society, there are many myths about emotions. We're aware that some are outmoded, misguided, or flat-out false. Other myths, however, still feel true. Sadly, we use them to guide our behavior, sometimes with problematic results.

Take this quiz to discover if you may be at the mercy of your emotions due to your belief in one or more myths.

1. Negative emotions are . . .

    a. To be avoided at all costs. They simply drain our positivity.

    b. The product of a bad attitude. It's best to aspire to be consistently happy.

    c. Effective in helping us identify situations we want to change or areas in which we need to work on acceptance.

2. Changing my negative emotions . . .

    a. Means I am a fake, a poseur, a phony.

    b. Is important. Negativity always drains the soul.

    c. May or may not be useful. I should consider this further to figure out what's best for me.

3. When I feel an emotion, it is best for me to . . .

    a. Trust and act on that emotion immediately. Why waste time?

    b. Find out how others feel and try my best to align with those feelings. It's best to stay in the groove with my family, friends, and coworkers.

    c. Pay attention to the emotion. The better I understand it, the better equipped I am to consider both my short-term and long-term goals.

4. My emotions are . . .

    a. Who I am—like it or not. I can't do anything about them, so I just roll with the feelings.

    b. Not to be trusted. Emotions can be obstacles that stand in the way of happiness.

    c. To be listened to, certainly, but are only one factor in making effective decisions.

5. If I don't express all emotions . . .

    a. The emotion will leak out at a moment of weakness and maybe result in unexpected problems.

b. Others will approve of me. No one wants to deal with an emotional friend, coworker, or loved one.

c. It may be evidence that I am gaining the ability to regulate and making good decisions about when and how to express my emotions.

6. If I feel a negative emotion . . .

    a. I could get stuck in it and feel this way for a long time (or even forever).

    b. It's a telltale indicator that my life is not going well. The last thing I need is for others to think I am flighty, unpredictable, or "crazy."

    c. I can determine if it is effective for me to feel this emotion—or if it benefits me to change it.

7. My emotions are . . .

    a. Why people love me.

    b. How others judge me.

    c. All mine. And I can decide what to do with them.

8. Being emotional means . . .

    a. I am passionate about life. I live without unnecessary restrictions, regardless of how my emotions may impact others.

    b. I am out of control. No one wants to hear about my feelings. It's best to always tamp them down.

    c. I am human.

9. Letting others know how I feel is . . .

    a. Always a good idea.

    b. Never a good idea.

    c. A choice. It's a decision I can make each time, based on the situation.

10. Controlling my emotions means . . .

    a. I am a robot. Living an emotion-free life isn't practical or healthy.

    b. I can effectively control how other people feel about me.

    c. I can decide how to act depending on the wide range of scenarios I face each day.

Scoring

Total the number of As, Bs, and Cs. If you scored:

- ☐ **Mostly As:** Emotional myths are getting in your way. You have been taught that emotions must always be trusted and expressed. Believing this myth may keep you from regulating your emotions in a healthy way.

- ☐ **Mostly Bs:** You may be relinquishing your control to others. Always trusting friends, coworkers, loved ones, or even strangers to decide what your beliefs should be isn't healthy. Fear of judgment from others may be limiting you. Learning to identify your own feelings will be key in learning to regulate your emotions.

- ☐ **Mostly Cs:** Yay! You are on your way! Sometimes, it's beneficial to feel our emotions openly. And, other times, it may be helpful or productive to regulate those emotions. Understanding this can be important, especially during difficult or complex times.

States of Mind

Dialectical behavior therapy (DBT), an evidence-based psychotherapy that improves emotional regulation, posits that we have three states of mind:

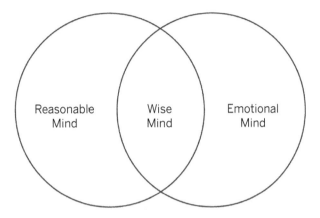

Reasonable Mind is the logical, rule- and task-oriented part of our psyche. It's essential, of course, to help us be good citizens or reliable workers.

But when our reasonable mind is not balanced by our Emotional and Wise Minds, we are ruled solely by facts, rules, and procedures.

Would you want to face a judge who did not take mitigating circumstances into consideration when issuing a ruling? Stole a loaf of bread? Cut off their hand!

Reasonable mind is great for solving math equations, but not always great for our relationships.

Wise Mind reflects the savvy, prudence, and wisdom that each of us builds over the years, shaped by our daily lives and what we learn from them.

It is the ability to balance reason and emotion, but adds more: intuition, foresight, and "what really matters."

We all possess Wise Mind, but some of us have a harder time accessing it than others. It can take practice.

It is the part of each person that can experience "truth."

This is where we want to be when making important decisions.

Emotional Mind is propelled by feelings, moods, and urges.

When the Emotional Mind is not balanced by our Reasonable and Wise Minds, our feelings are entirely in control.

Our whole state of mind can swing from "Gimme more!" to "Make it stop!" and back again. Nothing matters except our immediate desires and urges.

Being in full-bore Emotional Mind can lead to some risky situations. And it's not the place we want to be when making vital choices that can impact our lives, our jobs, and our relationships.

CONTINUED»

Emotional Mind is ruled by urges. How do you tend to act when you are in Emotional Mind? What kind of choices do you make? What is the impact on people around you?

Angry most of the time sometimes
numb they don't want to talk to me.

Reasonable Mind is ruled by logic and facts, undiluted by emotion or wisdom. How do you tend to act when in reasonable mind? What kind of choices do you make? What is the impact on people around you?

they don't understand me flew upset
straight forward

Wise Mind requires both reason and emotion. It taps the wisdom within us that helps us avoid acting impulsively. It is the state of mind we want to be in when making crucial decisions. How do you tend to act when in Wise Mind? What kind of choices do you make? What is the impact on people around you?

Very rational people love me I'm
funny

Beyond the Book: Accessing Wise Mind

Remember when we talked about mindfulness on page 22? This state of being, the awareness that arises through paying attention to the present moment without judgment, is the path to accessing Wise Mind. Some people know they are in Wise Mind when they feel a sense of calm in the center of their body. Others feel it in their "third eye," defined by Hindus as the *Ajna* chakra, in which we feel intuition, clarity, and internal bliss. Others describe a sense of intellectual bliss. In whichever way you feel it, you'll only recognize it when you attain it.

Try this meditation for 5 to 10 minutes to assess how you might experience Wise Mind.

1. Sit in a comfortable position, and take a few gentle deep breaths.

2. Continue breathing (always a good idea!). While breathing in, notice the slight pause at the top of the inhale.

3. On the out breath, notice the slight pause at the bottom of the exhale.

4. At each pause, allow yourself to feel the stillness within the pause. In that pause, you may find the feeling of being in Wise Mind, the place where we humans plot out our most assured, thoughtful, and effective actions—and live our best lives.

Explore How Moods, Emotions, and Behaviors Are Linked

Behaviors, moods, and emotions can be strongly linked. Sometimes they are inseparable. And they can cause us to get snagged into a seemingly unbreakable, self-defeating cycle.

Ever feel low and depressed for an extended period? The sadness is an emotion, of course, but if we don't recognize and respond to it, it can expand into mood. And that can fuel a behavior. We may feel so sad that it makes us tired, so we may try to avoid daily activities, putting our job or our relationships at risk. The behavior could take its toll on our health, too, if we respond by "self-medicating" with unhealthy food, alcohol, or drugs.

We may not even know that the original emotion is feeding the mood that becomes the behavior, which in turn strengthens the emotion. Yeah, it can be a vicious cycle. If we are honest with ourselves, we know that we don't always cope in healthy ways. That's because, even when we acknowledge such emotions, we don't truly understand them. And we don't yet know that we can regulate them by tapping our Wise Mind.

That's why we're here: As you get more familiar with your feelings and the situations that help create them, the more ways you can turn them around and even apply them to growing stronger. That's where we are going to focus next.

The Feelings Chart

Being able to identify feelings starts with increasing your emotional vocabulary. This feelings chart offers a number of descriptive words that you can choose from to describe the emotion or emotions you are feeling. You can run down this list and choose the emotion that feels most valid at any given time. You aren't limited by the words in the chart, so if you know you feel something that isn't listed, use your own word!

Amused	Embarrassed	Intimate	Sad
Angry	Energetic	Irritated	Satisfied
Anxious	Excited	Jealous	Scared
Apathetic	Faithful	Joyful	Secure
Appreciated	Foolish	Lonely	Selfish
Ashamed	Frustrated	Loving	Serene
Aware	Furious	Mad	Skeptical
Bewildered	Guilty	Miserable	Sleepy
Bored	Hateful	Nurturing	Stupid
Cheerful	Helpless	Peaceful	Thankful
Confident	Hopeful	Pensive	Thoughtful
Confused	Hostile	Playful	Trusting
Content	Hurt	Powerful	Valuable
Creative	Important	Proud	Vibrant
Critical	Inadequate	Rage	Weak
Daring	Inferior	Rejected	Worthwhile
Delightful	Insecure	Relaxed	
Depressed	Insignificant	Respected	
Discouraged	Intelligent	Responsive	

Try checking in with this list each day to develop more self-awareness about your emotions. Not only will this help you understand how they fluctuate, it will equip you with the right language to pinpoint any distressing emotions that you wish to regulate as you work through this book.

Observing the Parts
of Your Emotions

These are the five basic ways we experience an emotion:

1. **Prompting event:** This is the event that sets off the emotional experience in the first place. It's something that occurs right before an emotion starts. Some people call these "triggers." They can be external (something that happens outside of you in your environment) or internal (your own thoughts or behaviors).

2. **Thoughts:** What you are thinking as you experience an emotion (for example, "I suck," "I can't stand this," or "This is so cool!")

3. **Feelings:** The common name or label we give an emotion (sadness, joy, anger, etc.)

4. **Body sensations:** How your body responds (tension, butterflies in the stomach, clenched teeth, etc.)

5. **Action urges:** Impulses spurred by the emotion (to punch someone in the nose, to run away, to give someone a big hug, or to step on someone's cupcake).

The worksheet on page 43 can be used to log the emotions you feel in varying situations to start increasing your self-awareness. At the end of each day, choose four or five of the strongest emotions you felt during the day. Review the five ways we experience an emotion and fill out the chart for each emotion felt as best as you can. The more you do this, the easier it will become.

PROMPTING EVENT	
THOUGHTS	
FEELINGS	
BODY SENSATIONS	
ACTION URGES	

Behavioral Activation

Behavioral activation is a strategy for combating negative emotions and creating positive ones. You can choose to engage in activities that make you feel a sense of achievement or enjoyment, whether or not you feel like it. For example, you can choose to exercise even when your emotions tell you to stay in bed. You can decide to go out with friends even though you want to stay home and hide. This is contrary to mood-dependent behavior, shown here:

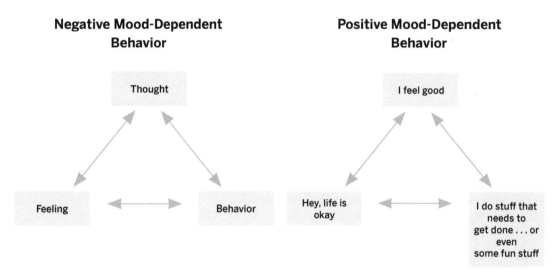

As illustrated, negative emotions, like the sadness associated with depression, can sap our motivation and prevent us from engaging in activities that might cause us to feel happy or attain a sense of achievement. Doing these activities anyway can result in a reduction of sadness because you are doing something pleasurable or necessary. Of course, it isn't always easy to do. But the payoffs can be great! .

Charting your engagement in the behavioral-activation activity that follows can show you the impact your choices are having on your mood. In the first column, record the activity you will engage in as part of this strategy. Then, using the rating chart, rate your negative emotions *before* and *after* the activity. Do the same with your level of pleasure and/or achievement. Be sure to balance tasks that need to be done with pleasurable activities that simply make you feel good. When choosing activities that must get done, try to pick activities that are manageable rather than tasks that feel like you need to move a mountain to even get them started. And when choosing pleasurable activities, remember to be especially mindful when doing the activity. That means paying attention to the activity to wring out as much pleasure from it as possible and to let go of feelings of guilt or thoughts that you don't deserve to have fun when you are "supposed" to be feeling sad or depressed.

Activities can be as simple as taking a shower or doing the dishes when you don't feel like it. Those are tasks that that simply need to be done. Pleasurable activities can be as simple as drinking a cup of tea or watching a movie.

RATING CHART

NONE	MINI-MAL	SLIGHT	MILD	MOD-ERATE	MUCH	HIGHER	HIGH	VERY HIGH	EXTREME
1	2	3	4	5	6	7	8	9	10

ACTIVITY	NEGATIVE EMOTION	PLEASURE	ACHIEVEMENT
	Before: .... After:	Before: .... After:	Before: .... After: ....
	Before: .... After:	Before: .... After:	Before: .... After: ....
	Before: .... After:	Before: .... After:	Before: .... After: ....

CONTINUED»

ACTIVITY	NEGATIVE EMOTION	PLEASURE	ACHIEVEMENT
	Before:	Before:	Before: ....
	....	....	....
	....	....	....
	After:	After:	After: ....
	....	....	....
	....	....	....

Beyond the Book: Taking Care of Your Mind by Taking Care of Your Body

Taking care of your body helps take care of your mind. The PLEASE skill from dialectical behavior therapy (DBT) can help you remember to do this. Here's what the acronym stands for:

- PL: Treat physical illness. See a doctor when needed, and take your prescribed medications.

- E: Balance your eating. Eat regularly throughout the day, and eat neither too much nor too little for your needs.

- A: Avoid mood-altering drugs. Keep away from alcohol (or use with moderation) and do not take nonprescribed drugs.

- S: Balance your sleep. Get enough sleep and stick to a consistent sleep schedule.

- E: Get plenty of exercise. Even if you are not running marathons, do some sort of physical movement every day.

This is the stuff Mom always bugged us about. Mom was right. Yay, moms!

Recognize and Accept Your Emotions

It makes sense that we want to avoid negative emotions. They are distinctly unpleasant. But attempting to avoid unpleasant emotions can backfire on us, causing us to feel them more frequently or more intensely. When we are willing to accept an emotion rather than reject it, it allows us to come to terms with reality and the inevitability of pain in life.

Why would we want to do this? Accepting negative emotions allows us to live life more completely. We can adopt more effective emotional-regulation strategies. Negative emotions are going to happen, whether or not we want them to. So, even if we don't like the idea of them, recognizing and accepting negative emotions are vital to a successful life and to emotional regulation.

If our goal is to simply to avoid negative emotions, we sometimes turn to ineffective or even dangerous ways of coping, for example:

* Alcohol or drugs

* Avoidance, or "hiding" from life

* Ruminating: becoming so focused on eluding bad feelings that we become obsessed with them

* Worrying: becoming so focused on trying to solve possible problems that we think about them ad nauseum

Habituation, or growing accustomed to feeling emotions, can make specific emotions less frightening. It can allow us the space we need to make more thoughtful choices and feel our emotions in a more effective way.

The exercises on the following pages will help you to better understand how and why certain emotions appear, and to come to terms with difficult feelings rather than being over-whelmed or trying to avoid them.

Recognizing Emotions: Your Tells

Have you ever played poker? If so, you might know what a "tell" is: that telltale shift in a player's behavior or demeanor that can tip off their opponent about what's in their hand. It might be the rubbing of the forehead or wide-open eyes or a barely discernable sigh. If a player observes and understands the meaning of another player's tell, they can gain an advantage.

Our emotions can work the same way. If we can recognize how and why emotions appear, we can learn to accept and manage them. So, pick up your cards. It's time to learn to identify your own emotional tells. Here's an example:

When I feel *anxious*, it is *because my boss gives me a look*.

        emotion   prompting event

My thought is *"I am going to get fired,"* my body feels *tense*,

               thought   body sensation

and I want to *run to the bathroom and cry*.

               action urge

After I feel this emotion, I notice that I *feel embarrassed and angry at myself*.

                              aftereffect of the emotion

Now it's your turn: Fill out these two prompts to discover your emotional tells.

When I feel _____, it is because _____ has happened.

               emotion   prompting event

My thought is _____, my body feels _____,

               thought   body sensation

and I want to _____.

               action urge

After I feel this emotion, I notice that I _____.

                       aftereffects of the emotion

Accepting Difficult Feelings

Here are some questions to ask yourself about feelings you don't necessarily want to accept to increase your self-awareness and your ability to accept difficult feelings:

What is the feeling you are finding hard to accept?

_____

_____

What is making you reluctant to accept this feeling?

_____

_____

_____

_____

Keeping in mind what you've learned about emotional acceptance, what are the pros and cons of accepting this feeling?

_____

_____

_____

_____

What might be different if you were able to accept this feeling?

_____

_____

_____

_____

Drop the Rope:
A Method for Accepting Feelings

Pretend you are playing tug-of-war. Your nemesis is Dwayne "The Rock" Johnson. You know him—handsome, charming, and muscled all over. Between you and The Rock is a scary pit. As near as you can tell, it's bottomless. If you lose this battle, into the pit you go. It's deep and dark, and heaven knows what awful creatures are hiding in there.

You don't want to end up in that pit. So you pull and pull and pull with all your might. The harder you pull, however, the harder The Rock pulls. And with each pull, you draw closer and closer to the edge of the pit.

How else can you stay out of the pit? You drop the rope, of course! The phrase "dropping the rope" means:

1. Stopping the useless fighting.

2. Accepting the feeling.

3. Eluding the dangers of ineffective coping.

What feeling do you need to "drop the rope" on? _____

Dropping the rope requires mindfulness of the emotion you are experiencing. First, rate the level of intensity of the feeling on a scale of 0 to 10 and record it here: _____.
Then, try this:

1. Step back and notice the feeling.

2. Let go of judgments about the feeling.

3. Notice your body sensations.

4. Practice being willing to accept the unwanted feeling.

5. Imagine your feelings on the car of a train, just passing by.

6. Notice any action urges you might have without acting on them.

7. Remind yourself of times when you have not felt this feeling.

8. Practice completely accepting the feeling, maybe even loving it a little.

After you have taken these steps, rate the level of intensity of the feeling again and record it here: _____.
What did you notice about this experience? Record your thoughts on the following page.

_____

_____

_____

_____

_____

Beyond the Book:
Riding the Wave of Emotion

Often, it is helpful to discover that emotions come and go. Just like a wave, an emotion will reach its peak and then retreat, easing into its ebb. Here are some guidelines for practicing "riding the wave":

1. Step back and notice the emotion.

2. Allow the emotion to rise.

3. Allow the emotion to fall.

4. Don't try to fight or suppress the emotion.

5. Don't try to hold on to the emotion.

6. Breathe into the emotion.

7. Relax into the emotion.

8. Ride the wave.

Unearth Root Causes

As you learned when we talked about acceptance, nonacceptance (or suppression of thoughts and feelings) can lead to them sticking around and even intensifying.

Try this out: Take a full minute and conjure in your mind a fluffy pink unicorn. It is so, so very fluffy! Got the image in place? Good! Now, for the next minute, whatever you do, don't think of that fluffy, fluffy pink unicorn. Just don't!

I'll bet you couldn't think of much of anything besides that unicorn. And you probably got annoyed with yourself because you couldn't *not* think about it. This silly example is representative of how avoidance of thoughts and feelings works.

Here's the main idea: Difficult thoughts, feelings, and events are just a part of life. There's simply no way around that. Aiming to avoid those feelings can be ineffective, futile, and even dangerous! And when we do avoid them, we feel relief, for a tiny window of time. And our brains say, "Whew, dodged that bullet!" So we avoid even more.

As we know, avoidance emboldens that fluffy unicorn of difficult thoughts and feelings to stick around even more! Maybe we stop going to certain places because they are where we thought of the fluffy pink unicorn. Maybe we avoid the people who remind us of that critter.

And as we try harder and harder to avoid those difficult thoughts and feelings, we miss out on all kinds of positive things about life. Or perhaps we don't take care of tasks that need to be accomplished, and find ourselves in big messes as a result.

On the following pages, you'll find some exercises to help you understand the cycle of avoidance and how to better navigate your worries and ruminations.

The Cycle of Avoidance

Avoiding situations, thoughts, and feelings that trigger negative emotions can provide relief in the short term. However, in the future, when faced with difficult events, our brain will scream even louder at us to avoid them. Take a look at this diagram:

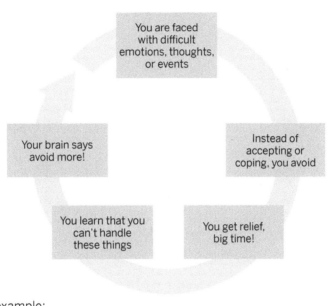

Here's a real-life example:

CONTINUED»

What are some of your cycles of avoidance? Record them here:

Prompting event

....

....

....

Avoidance behavior

....

....

....

Relief-based thought and feeling

....

....

....

Lesson learned from avoidance

....

....

....

What urges do you experience now?

....

....

....

Worry and Rumination

Worry is thinking about problems that might happen. It goes hand in hand with anxiety. Rumination, meanwhile, is when worry turns into repetitive thinking about the past. It is usually associated with depression.

You might think, "Hey, at least I'm thinking about these things. That won't lead to avoidance!" But it often does. When you worry about things you can do nothing about, some small part of your brain thinks you are actually doing something about the problem. When we obsessively chew on the past, we can actually think we are taking action that can change the past. We all know that's impossible, but our brains tend to do it anyway.

Helpful worry and rumination, of course, can lead to the resolution of an issue. But taken to extreme, it is a painful waste of time. Use the space below to write about your own relationship with worry and rumination.

Now, take a look at the decision tree on the following page to help you think through constructive action you can take the next time you find yourself caught in worry or rumination.

CONTINUED»

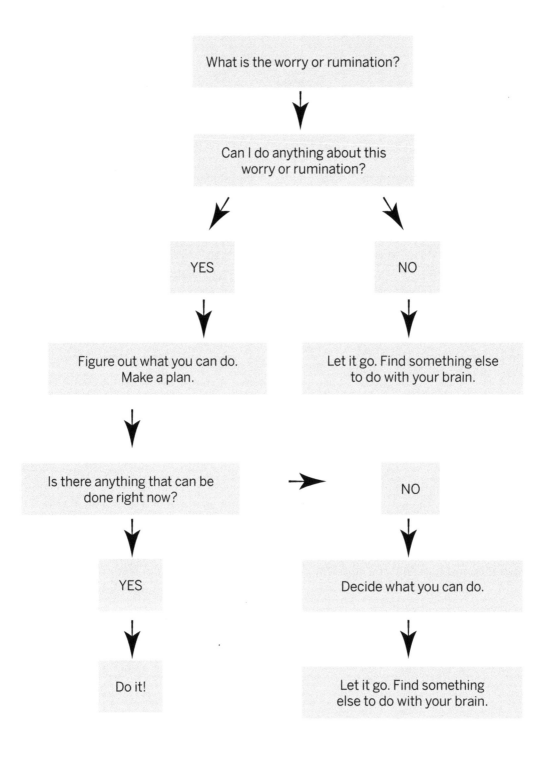

What is the worry or rumination?

Can I do anything about this worry or rumination?

YES

NO

Figure out what you can do. Make a plan.

Let it go. Find something else to do with your brain.

Is there anything that can be done right now?

NO

YES

Decide what you can do.

Do it!

Let it go. Find something else to do with your brain.

Now practice better navigating your worries and ruminations by answering the following questions.

What worry or rumination can you do something about right now?

....

....

What can you do about it?

....

....

Now, put this book down right now and do it! What worry or rumination can you do something about, but not right this minute?

....

....

What can you do?

....

....

When will you do it?

....

....

Make a written commitment to yourself that you will do it, and do it when you say you will do it.

....

....

What worry or rumination can you do nothing about? What else can you do with your brain?

....

....

Make a written commitment to yourself that you will engage in this process the next time you worry or ruminate.

....

Beyond the Book: Scheduling Worry Time

Having a hard time letting go of rumination or worries? Here's a strategy to postpone them:

1. **Create a specific "worry time."** Make an appointment with yourself. Choose a set time and place every day for worrying. It should not be close to bedtime. Let's say from 2 to 2:20 p.m. at your desk. During worry time, you will be allowed to worry about whatever you choose to worry about, but only for that established period of time.

2. **Write down your worries.** You can use a pad of paper, the back of an envelope, or even your smartphone. Tell yourself you will only worry about them during worry time.

3. **Go over your list of worries during "worry time."** Take out your worry list and focus on it. You may find that your worries seem less important or easier to solve when you sit and focus on them with a clear mind. If you do not have enough worries to fill the time, simply go about your day. Or you may find that you're actually writing down action steps to ease those worries. Woo-hoo!

Before You Move On

A lot was accomplished in this chapter! You've learned all about understanding your emotions and increasing your self-awareness. You've ascertained how emotion-related myths can get in your way. You've been introduced to the different states of mind and why the Wise Mind is the state to strive for. You've grown your "feelings vocabulary" and exposed yourself to the power of behavioral activation. You've been reminded about taking care of your body to take care of your mind and emotions, and you've gathered the strength to avert avoidance, worry, and rumination. Look at you go!

Takeaways

Let's focus on some key takeaways:

- Wise Mind is available to you, and mindfulness is the path to get there.

- Understanding and identifying your behaviors, moods, and feelings—and how they are linked—is a crucial step toward mastering emotional regulation.

- Trying to suppress and avoid emotions can only make them stronger and tougher to cope with.

- The cycle of avoidance increases negative feelings. While worrying or ruminating may convince you that you are taking action toward solving a problem, it is actually just a way of sidestepping reality.

Next Steps

- Get active and avoid avoiding!

- Identify and challenge those emotional myths.

- Strive for the Wise Mind.

- "Drop the rope" to accept your feelings and stay out of the pit of despair.

- Confront your cycles of avoidance.

CHAPTER FOUR

Managing Your Emotions

In this chapter, you will engage in more exercises and learn tips and tricks for managing emotions. You'll do the detective work of analyzing behavior and identifying triggers that set off behaviors and emotions. You'll also learn how to respond in a deliberate and measured way, rather than immediately reacting to triggering situations. You'll learn how to trick your nervous system into being less reactive. And you'll practice how to catch and reframe negative thoughts so you can change your feelings. It's a lot, but it's totally doable!

Identify Your Triggers

Knowing what sets off strong emotions can be really helpful in managing them. An emotional trigger is a memory, experience, or event that sparks an emotional reaction. Knowing your triggers is a key component of managing emotions. After all, if you know what sets off a reaction, you can predict and manage that reaction.

Everyone has certain emotional triggers, although they can look different for each person. Even your own emotion or behavior can be a trigger for more emotions and behaviors. To gain some insight into your emotional triggers, we are going to look at little slices of time in a very detailed way. From those little slices of life, you will pull out the elements that set you off and create problem behaviors and emotions for you—your triggers. You'll learn all kinds of ways to manage these triggers throughout this chapter and the rest of the book.

One tool we'll tap is called a behavior chain analysis. Think of this as being a detective, a behavioral Sherlock Holmes. Our case: Scrutinizing the elements that can cause a behavior, just like Sherlock searching for the clues to solve a crime (not that having an emotion is a crime, of course). We need Sherlock's help on this because, after all, if it were easy, you would have figured it out already. The game's afoot, Watson!

Common Emotional Triggers

Here are some common triggers to emotion. Keep them in mind or refer to this list as you are analyzing your behavior. Circle the ones that are triggers for you and add others that aren't listed in the space provided.

Abandonment	Feeling like "the bad guy"	Lectures	Scary circumstances
Being ignored and/or overlooked	Feeling taken for granted	Loneliness	Shameful experiences
Betrayal	Frustration	Manipulation	Small gatherings
Confinement (feeling trapped)	Getting left out of something	Misunderstandings	Tardiness
Criticism	Inability to speak up and/or be honest	Not knowing what's going to happen	Uncertainty
Disconnection		Overwhelm	Unfairness
Disrespect		Plans falling through	Unfamiliar settings, tasks, and/or people
Dramatic people	Jealousy	Powerlessness	Unpreparedness
Embarrassing situations	Lack of affection	Rejection	Vulnerability
Envy	Lack of attention	Reminders of trauma	Words falling on deaf ears
Exclusion	Lack of love and/or support	Risks (feeling unsafe)	
Feeling dispensable	Large events		

....

....

....

....

....

....

Creating a Behavior Chain

A behavior chain shows a sequence of emotions, events, thoughts, and other factors to better understand their effect on a person's behavior. It involves consideration of the following things:

Emotion and Behavior: What was the emotion? Was there a behavior that occurred because of this emotion?

Prompting Event: What was the event that set the emotion off? This could be something that happened in your environment, a thought, a feeling, or an action taken by someone else.

Vulnerabilities: Was there anything that happened 24 to 48 hours prior to the prompting event that made you feel vulnerable?

Links: These are thoughts, feelings, actions you took, body sensations, and people and things in your environment. What were the links between the prompting event and the behavior/emotion?

Consequences: How did your emotions and actions affect you immediately? How did they affect you later? What were the short-term and long-term consequences?

Now, let's put the answers to those questions into a chain. Here is an example of a person who feels angry at their partner, Taylor, after they canceled dinner plans.

	THINGS TO CONSIDER	EXAMPLE NOTES
Vulnerabilities	Any triggers in the past 24 to 48 hours that made you feel vulnerable. Such as: ☐ Physical illness, injury, pain ☐ Fatigue, hunger ☐ Stressful events	*I hadn't slept well, I was worn out from a stressful week at work, and I had a headache. Taylor and I haven't been out much lately, and I was really looking forward to a fun evening out.*
Prompting Event	The event, thought, or feeling that set the problem emotion off.	*Taylor was not only late coming over, but also wanted to cancel the restaurant reservation and just watch Netflix and chill.*

CONTINUED»

	THINGS TO CONSIDER	EXAMPLE NOTES
Links	The links between the prompting event, thought, or feeling and the problem emotion.	*I thought, "What? Are you kidding?" I was a little bit hurt at first, but then I was really angry. It was super noticeable. Taylor apologized and said we could do it another time soon. My body was tense and tight, and my jaw was clenched. Taylor kept trying to joke with me and be loving, but I was too upset to respond.*
Problem Behavior or Emotion	What emotions and/or behaviors occurred because of this emotion?	*I stayed super angry, even though I had done something similar last week when we were supposed to go out. I didn't talk about my sadness and disappointment that our plans were broken. I just stayed quiet and seethed.*
Consequences	What were the short- and long-term consequences of your emotions and actions?	*We ordered pizza and sat really far away from each other while we watched a movie. It was a lousy night. I had to apologize the next day because I felt guilty that I wasn't as understanding as Taylor had been when I had canceled plans the previous week. I think if this keeps happening, it may be really bad for our relationship.*

Now it's your turn. Bring to mind a strong emotion you experienced recently. Write down your notes in the blank column on the next page to see the sequence of events that led to your emotion and how that affected your behavior.

	THINGS TO CONSIDER	MY NOTES
Prompting Event	Any triggers in the past 24 to 48 hours that made you feel vulnerable, such as: ☐ Physical illness, injury, pain ☐ Fatigue, hunger ☐ Stressful events	
Prompting Event, Thought, or Feeling	The event, thought, or feeling that set the problem emotion off.	
Links	The links between the prompting event, thought, or feeling and the problem emotion.	
Problem Behavior or Emotion	What emotions and/or behaviors occurred because of this emotion?	
Consequences	What were the short- and long-term consequences of your emotions and actions?	

What Are Your Triggers?

Considering all the information you gleaned from the previous two exercises, look again at the list of triggers on page 62. Remember: If nothing on the list seems to fit, you can add your own. The two to five triggers I have identified are:

....

....

Keep these in mind as you do the other exercises in this book.

Make Space Between Your Reaction and Your Response

Remember when we talked about reflexive versus reflective behavior on page 14? This is where that comes into play. In managing emotions, there are a couple of different scenarios:

1. **The life-threatening crisis.** Are you being chased by drooling zombies, grizzly bears, or murderous clowns? Those are all absolutely crisis situations. Should you react impulsively? Heck, yeah! React *all* you want and get the heck out of there! *Your choice: Reacting in an impulsive and immediate way.*

2. **Everything else.** In most scenarios, we can pause, even very briefly, and choose a considered, measured response. It can take practice. Taking time to craft a deliberate plan of action in response to emotional triggers is an attainable skill. Just so long as there are no zombies. *Your choice: Responding in a measured and deliberate way.*

It is critically important to remember that the limbic system within our brains still often reacts as if our lives were being threatened when there is absolutely no risk. Learning how to override the fight-flight-freeze response is vital in managing emotions.

Responding versus Reacting

When faced with triggers, we can choose different ways to cope. Look at the pairs of words in each row. Choose one word from either column A or column B that describes your usual experience in dealing with triggers for each row.

COLUMN A	COLUMN B
Deliberate	Impulsive
Delayed	Immediate
Mindful	Unmindful
Wise Mind	Emotional Mind
You are in control	Situation is in control
Not a crisis	"Sure feels like a crisis"
Resisting immediate action urges	Acting on immediate action urges

You may have guessed that column A is about **responding in a measured and deliberate way** to emotional triggers and column B is about **reacting in an impulsive and immediate way**. Responding is the way to go when emotional regulation is desired.

If you chose more As than Bs, good for you! You are on the road to mastering your response instead of instantly reacting. If you chose more Bs than As, don't sweat it. The remaining exercises in this chapter provide specific skills you can use to be more measured and intentional when faced with emotional triggers.

Pros and Cons

This exercise is intended to be done in advance of a triggering situation when you are in Wise Mind. A "pros and cons" list is intended to be a tip sheet from your Wise Mind on the preferred response to a triggering situation.

Here is an example: Your boss, yet again, has asked you to stay late without any advance notice. You already paid for a nonrefundable yoga class right after work. You started doing yoga to help regulate your emotions and manage stress (much of it caused by the boss!), and missing this class is really going to harsh your mellow. Your instant reaction: Give your two weeks' notice *right now*. The problem: The rent is due and jobs don't grow on trees.

	PROS	CONS
Reacting to the triggering situation	☐ I am a valuable employee, and I don't deserve this! I quit! ☐ "Take this job and shove it" would feel really good—and mighty country-retro-cool to sing on my way out the door. ☐ The boss would get the message and feel some pain in trying to replace me. That'll show him! ☐ Time for yoga!	☐ Um . . . no job means no money. ☐ I actually like my job most days. I could take or leave my boss, but I enjoy my coworkers and consider them friends. ☐ Um . . . no money is really a big problem. ☐ My partner would be really mad at me for quitting without having another job lined up. ☐ Next job might not be as good if I am trying to get one really quickly. ☐ Um . . . how am I gonna pay for yoga?

	PROS	CONS
Responding to the triggering situation	☐ I would feel mature and competent for handling the situation like an adult. ☐ I could probably ask for a quick meeting with my boss to figure out other ways to get help without me having to stay without some advance warning. ☐ Dealing with this in a professional way might show I am ready for a raise and a promotion. ☐ My partner wouldn't be mad at me for quitting. Like last time. That was ugly. ☐ I wouldn't have to look for a new job.	☐ My boss might keep asking me to stay late unless I figure out how to talk to them. ☐ I wouldn't get the satisfaction of telling my boss off.

CONTINUED»

Now, you give this a try with one of your triggering situations. Remember to engage Wise Mind!

	PROS	CONS
Reacting to the triggering situation	....	....
	....	....
	....	....
	....	....
	....	....
	....	....
	....	....
	....	....
	....	....
	....	....
	....	....
	....	....
Responding to the triggering situation	....	....
	....	....
	....	....
	....	....
	....	....
	....	....
	....	....
	....	....
	....	....
	....	....
	....	....

The STOP Skill

Marsha Linehan, the creator of dialectical behavior therapy (DBT), recommends the STOP skill for putting some space between a trigger and your response. It works like this:

1. **S**top. Seriously, stop! Don't move! Freeze for a moment before the urge to react takes over.

2. **T**ake a step back. Take a step back either physically or mentally. Take a few deep breaths. Do not let your urge to react take over.

3. **O**bserve. Observe and describe what is really happening. No judgments, assumptions, or interpretations. Just the facts, please.

4. **P**roceed mindfully. Ask your Wise Mind what the best response might be. What outcome will you feel best about tomorrow or next week?

What are the triggering situations when you might need to practice the STOP skill?

....

....

....

....

Make a plan and jot it down here. If you need more room, use a piece of paper or a computer document.

....

....

....

....

You might even make a copy of the STOP steps and post it on your bathroom mirror and your refrigerator as a useful reminder to practice this skill.

....

....

....

Beyond the Book: Paced Breathing

Paced breathing is a great way to get the parasympathetic nervous system online when faced with a triggering situation. Our autonomic nervous system has two responses: 1) the sympathetic nervous system, which is associated with the fight-flight-freeze response, and 2) the parasympathetic nervous system, associated with the "rest and digest" response.

Inhaling activates the sympathetic nervous system. It prepares us for action. Exhaling activates the parasympathetic nervous system, which calms us down. The trick here is to spend more time exhaling than inhaling so your body gets to slow down, calm down, and relax. Let's give it a go!

Here's the basic technique:

1. Inhale for a count of two to four seconds.

2. Exhale for a count of four to six seconds.

3. Continue for a few minutes or as long as desired.

Find the combination that works for you, making sure to exhale longer than you inhale. Here are some things to keep in mind as you go:

- Breathe in slowly through your nose, letting your chest and lower belly expand.

- Breathe out slowly through your mouth, pursing your lips and making a *swoosh* sound. (You don't have to *swoosh* if there are other people, of course—unless they are *swooshing,* too.)

- If your mind wanders, gently redirect your focus back to the counting and breathing.

- For maximum calming effects, try to slow your breathing down to five or six breath cycles per minute.

This breathing exercise works even better when you practice in advance of triggering situations, because you will have trained yourself to be able to activate the relaxation response more readily.

Shift Your Focus

Mindfulness is all about observing and responding to your thoughts and emotions, rather than them being in charge of you. For many of us, our minds are all over the place. The good news is that you can build the muscle of mindfulness. Each time you bring yourself back to the task at hand, you pump up this muscle. The goal of mindfulness is simple; the execution is what takes some practice and hard work.

Think of the mind as an untrained puppy. When we engage the puppy, we gently reel the pooch back in to the tasks we want it to do. It's the same process, basically, with the mind. Every time we bring the mind back to the mindfulness task we have chosen, we are training the mind. We don't want the mind to fetch our slippers, though; we want it to be more focused and aware.

When distractions arise, thank the mind and return to the task at hand. Again and again and again. Think of this as the bicep curl of mindfulness. Every time you do it, your ability to decide where to place your awareness gets stronger.

The remaining exercises in this section will help you do just this. You'll find a tracking log so that you can make mindfulness a part of your daily routine, a range of ideas for helping you approach negative experiences more mindfully, and a grounding body-scan practice to help you shift your focus to the present moment.

Beyond the Book:
Mindfulness Cheat Sheet

Here's a quick and dirty checklist for attaining mindfulness:

1. **Identify what you will focus on.** You can focus on your breath, the sounds around you, a pencil, pretty much anything inside or outside of you.

2. **Remind yourself that distractions will arise.** Every time you bring yourself back to the mindfulness activity, you are building your mindfulness muscle. Yay distractions! Who knew they could be good for us?

3. **Decide how long you will practice.** Setting a timer is a great idea. You can do as little as a minute to start. Try to build your time as you gain more attentional control.

When your attention wanders, acknowledge the distraction, and gently bring your focus back. You may notice that your attention wanders in response to sounds, thoughts, judgments, body sensations (like itching), or that pair of flamenco dancers in the apartment upstairs. Notice them, then let them go, and return to the thing you are focusing on.

Remember, too, that there are plenty of apps for helping you practice mindfulness. See the resources on page 143 for some suggestions.

Build Your Mindfulness Muscle

To start training your brain to be more mindful, set a goal to practice daily, or at least a few times this week. Complete this log each day. If you'd like to continue this log after the week is up, you can do so in a notebook or computer document.

		OBSERVATIONS GLEANED FROM PRACTICE
Monday Date:	Did you practice? Y or N	
Tuesday Date:	Did you practice? Y or N	
Wednesday Date:	Did you practice? Y or N	
Thursday Date:	Did you practice? Y or N	
Friday Date:	Did you practice? Y or N	
Saturday Date:	Did you practice? Y or N	
Sunday Date:	Did you practice? Y or N	

Improve the Moment

The "improve the moment" skill is comprised of a menu of options you can use to shift your focus by making your negative experience a more positive one. Here are the options, which make up the acronym IMPROVE:

Imagery	Imagery can be used in many ways. You can imagine yourself in a peaceful, soothing place. You can imagine stress and painful emotions flowing out of you. You can even picture yourself coping extraordinarily well with whatever situation you find yourself in.
Meaning	Find meaning in the painful situation you face. Focus on whatever positives you can find in your current scenario. How can what you learn from this situation be used to help others?
Prayer	Prayer means different things to different people. You might view prayer as accessing Wise Mind or turning things over to something bigger than yourself. Perhaps you believe in a higher power. However you tap this skill, ask for the strength to bear the situation, not for the situation to magically disappear.
Relaxing actions	There are so many things that can bring a bit of relaxation to a difficult situation. Perhaps a few deep breaths? A walk, some yoga, or a nice bath? Relaxing activities can bring you to a better place to deal with current challenges, and at least they can't make things worse.
One thing in the moment	Bring a mindful focus to whatever you are doing in the moment. Notice when your mind starts to get caught up in painful thoughts about the past or fears for the future. Instead, focus intently on the task you currently need to perform.
Vacation	This doesn't mean packing your bags for Bermuda! It means to plan a brief respite from your current challenges. If you are going to take a one-hour breather from life, make sure you set a timer and commit to returning when the timer goes off. Now go have fun!
Encouragement	Sometimes, we all need some cheerleading. We can tell ourselves, "This is hard, but I can do it," "I am doing the best I can," "Go Team Me!" or "This, too, shall pass." The important part is to talk to yourself the way you would to someone you love.

When you feel an increase in negative emotions, refer to the IMPROVE options and complete the following log for the option chosen. Start by describing the situation that triggered the emotion(s) and identify the activity you will do or did. Use the table on page 76 for ideas around what activities you can use. Rate your level of distress *before* and *after* you engage in the activity.

	SITUATION	ACTIVITY USED	LEVEL OF DISTRESS BEFORE (0–10)	LEVEL OF DISTRESS AFTER (0–10)
Imagery				
Meaning				
Prayer				
Relaxing Action				
One thing in the moment				
Vacation				
Encouragement				

The Body Scan

Shifting focus with a body scan is a great idea because, no matter what, your body is always with you! The purpose is to tune in to your body, notice any sensations you're feeling without judgment, and ultimately become more accepting of what you feel. With patience, this can build your ability be fully present in your life and choose what you focus on.

This exercise can be as long or as short as you like. Here's how to do a body scan:

1. Sit in a comfortable position. When you are ready, close your eyes or find a place 12 to 18 inches in front of you to softly gaze upon.

2. Feel your weight on the chair, then feel your feet on the ground. Notice your toes. Where is your body touching the chair or the floor? Are those areas tense or relaxed?

3. Bring your hands together and rest them in your lap. How do they feel? Are they heavy or light? Warm or cool? Relaxed or tense?

4. Go back to your feet. How do they feel? Heavy or light? Warm or cool? Relaxed or tense?

5. Notice your calves. How do they feel?

6. Move to your knees and thighs. How do these parts of your body feel?

7. Move to your belly. Breathe in, letting your belly slowly fill with air, and then slowly breathe out.

8. Notice your fingertips. How do they feel? Move your attention up your arms, through your elbows, and up to your shoulders. How do these parts of your body feel? Heavy or light? Warm or cool? Relaxed or tense?

9. Move to your back. Notice how it feels. Warm or cool? Tense or relaxed?

10. Now notice your face. How does it feel?

11. Take a deep breath, and you're done!

Reframe Your Thoughts

When a triggering event happens, we tend to have an automatic thought about the event, often related to our past experiences or beliefs we carry around. This thought then has consequences, usually impacting our emotions and our behaviors.

Notice that the arrows go both ways in the following image. A negative feeling can cause a negative thought and a negative behavior can cause a negative feeling. Getting caught in patterns of negative emotion, thinking, and behavior can cause a whole lot of grief!

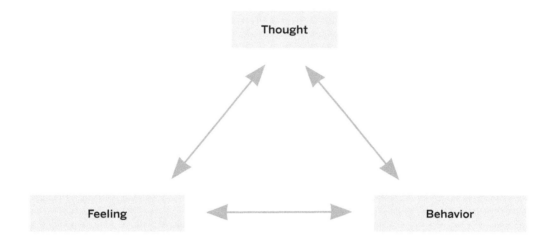

Reframing thoughts can help break this cycle. The first step is awareness. Acknowledge your thoughts, the feelings they create, and the consequences that occur. You'll do that in the following thought log.

In the rest of the chapter, you'll find other exercises to help you take this skill further, including how to catch negative thoughts, how to create new, helpful thoughts, and how to make these more automatic in the long term.

Thought Log

How we think often impacts how we feel. Keeping this log will help you see how your thoughts affect your feelings and actions. You can write about recent examples from your life if you wish to complete the activity now, or return to the log after events throughout the week. An example has been provided to help you get the hang of this.

EVENT	AUTOMATIC THOUGHT	CONSEQUENCE
Stuck in traffic.	*Why does this always happen to me? I'm never going to get to work.*	*Felt super frustrated. Went into work and was snappy and tense with my coworkers.*

Catching Negative Thoughts

Catching yourself having negative thoughts allows you to notice more about your thoughts and how they impact your emotions. It also allows you the chance to change those thoughts to more neutral or even more positive thoughts so that you can benefit by experiencing more neutral or positive emotions.

Deciding whether a thought is negative or not involves asking yourself a series of questions. Choose one of the thoughts from your thought log and apply these questions to it.

* Is this thought helpful?   **Y   N**

* Is this thought based on fact? In other words, do I have evidence to support this?   **Y   N**

* Am I caught up in negative thinking?   **Y   N**

* Am I ignoring the positive things in my life?   **Y   N**

* Is there an alternate explanation? In other words, could something else be true?   **Y   N**

* Is this a catastrophe?   **Y   N**

* Am I using "exaggerating" words, such as never, always, forever, need, should, must, can't, and every time?   **Y   N**

* Is this super important to my future? In other words, will I still think this is important a day, a week, or a year from now?   **Y   N**

Scoring

If you answered mostly no, that's good news, you are able to frame your thought in a neutral or positive way. The following exercises will still be useful to cement this ability with other thoughts you may have. If you answered yes more often than no, it is likely that this is a negative automatic thought. Don't worry. You can reframe it, as you'll learn next.

Reframing a Negative Thought

Identify a negative thought and ask yourself the following questions:

What else could be true?

_____

_____

_____

_____

If the worst did happen, what could I do to handle it? Who would help me?

_____

_____

_____

_____

What would people who care about me say about this thought? What would I say to a good friend who had this thought?

_____

_____

_____

_____

Based on your previous answer, what is your more helpful, effective thought?

_____

_____

_____

_____

Consolidating New Automatic Thoughts

In the previous exercise, you had the chance to create a new, more helpful effective thought. Now think about some of those thoughts that just pop right up all the time. Like perhaps, "I can't stand this." That thought often happens when we are doing something we don't like to do.

Obviously, we *can* stand it because we are still standing. So, a more effective automatic thought would be: "I don't like this, but I can stand it."

Now, bring to mind one of those unhelpful automatic thoughts that often pops up in your mind. Maybe you're in a meeting and tell yourself, "I'll sound like an idiot if I share my idea." Then, just as you did in the previous exercise, ask yourself, "What else could be true?" You might say, "They might not like my idea, but it's not senseless or foolish. It's well thought out." If the worst did happen (your boss actually calls you an idiot), what could you do to handle it? ("I could stand up for myself and ask not to be spoken to that way.") Who would help me? Well, in this case, human resources.

So, what's the more helpful, effective thought here? "They might not like my idea, but it's well thought out." Using this process, come up with four effective automatic thoughts for the negative ones that often pop up, and start turning to them instead.

Effective Automatic Thought 1

Effective Automatic Thought 2

Effective Automatic Thought 3

Effective Automatic Thought 4

Great job! You are on your way to more effective thinking!

Beyond the Book: Leaves in a Stream Mindfulness Exercise

Sometimes, certain thoughts can stick around longer than necessary. Here's a great way to take a moment of mindfulness and let thoughts go like leaves floating downstream.

1. Sit in a position that is comfortable for you to hold for a few minutes. Close your eyes.

2. Visualize yourself by a stream with leaves floating along on the gently flowing water.

3. Place each thought that enters your mind on one of the leaves and watch it float by. No matter whether the thoughts are, positive or negative, place each one on a leaf and watch it float away.

4. If you don't have any thoughts for a bit, just watch the stream. Sooner or later, you will have another thought.

5. Allow the stream to flow at its own pace. Don't rush it along simply to get rid of your thoughts. Allow the stream and the leaves to come and go at their own pace.

6. If you have judgments about this exercise, put those thoughts on leaves and let them float by. If you notice feelings, put thoughts about those feelings on leaves and let them float by.

7. If a leaf gets stuck, allow it to get stuck until it eventually floats by.

8. From time to time, you may get hooked by a thought and notice your attention has been distracted. This is to be expected. As soon as you realize this, place that thought on a leaf and let if float by.

9. Do this until you feel ready to go back to your usual day.

Before You Move On

In this chapter, you analyzed your behavior and identified triggers. You identified the pros and cons of reaction and response, and learned a few great tricks to help you pause before reacting. You've also explored how mindfulness can help you shift your focus. You even filled out a thought log, caught your negative thoughts, and learned to reframe them. You've also started to build some new automatic thoughts. Yay you!

Takeaways

Let's focus on some key takeaways:

- Knowing your triggers is a super-effective step in regulating emotions.

- Finding that space between reaction and response will help you regulate more often and more effectively.

- Shifting your focus helps you continue to find that space between an instant reaction and an effective response.

- Changing your thoughts can change your emotions and behaviors.

Next Steps

What's next?

- Practice analyzing situations to better identify your triggers.

- Prepare and review your pros and cons list so you can respond rather than react.

- Practice your mindfulness practice. They call it a practice for a reason. Practice!

- Remember to review those new thoughts you aim to make automatic.

- Give yourself a high five for making it this far.

Let's keep going!

CHAPTER FIVE

Conquering Negativity

In this chapter, you'll reduce negativity by participating in exercises and learning tips and tricks to conquer negative emotions—and maybe even use them to grow. You will learn to manage your inner critic, pump up your self-esteem, and strengthen your self-compassion. You'll get better at tempering strong emotions such as anger, shame, resentment, and jealousy. Our goal: Replace negativity with self-respect and zeal—and open up new opportunities for enjoying life.

Quiet Your Inner Critic

Almost all of us have an inner critic. For some, it is a tiny voice that gives helpful feedback when we have gone off course. If that's how your inner critic works, congratulations. However, for some of us, that inner critic is an angry and shaming figure with a high-powered megaphone.

Mind you, your inner critic probably once sounded like a friend—a tiny voice providing helpful, corrective feedback in a kind and caring way. Maybe you started to hear too much negative feedback from authority figures, or perhaps you were emotionally sensitive, so even a small amount of negative feedback resonated loudly. Whatever the case, over the years, your inner critic has likely grown louder and nastier and more self-defeating.

The irony is that as long as we judge ourselves harshly, we believe we are teaching ourselves new positive behaviors. Being critical assures we'll improve, right? Not really. In actuality, we are keeping ourselves mired in deeply damaging patterns of destructive self-judgment and negative emotions.

Put your inner critic on hold for a while, and let's learn more about where the voice comes from. And, no, you don't suck. Honest.

How Loud Is Your Inner Critic?

Everyone has an inner critic, but some are louder and more persuasive that others. It's time to discover how loud your inner critic is and how much power it holds. For each of the following statements, respond *rarely*, *sometimes*, or *frequently*.

	RARELY	SOMETIMES	FREQUENTLY
I second-guess my decisions.			
I feel terrible when I say "no."			
I do not like how I look, even when I make an effort with my appearance.			
I don't like to share my opinions.			
I compare myself with others and find myself wanting.			
I wonder what people would think if they *really* knew me.			
I judge myself.			
I worry about what others think of me.			
I replay my mistakes before I sleep.			
I replay conversations after they have happened to assess how I have messed up.			

Scoring

Give yourself 1 point for each statement you answered "rarely," 3 points for each statement you answered "sometimes," and 5 points for each statement you answered "frequently."
Total score: _____

- ☐ **1–23: Mild**. Your inner critic is more of a frenemy. It will be pretty easy to improve this relationship.

- ☐ **24–32: Moderate**. There's some work to be done here, but have faith. Some helpful tips and tricks are coming.

- ☐ **33–50: Severe**. Okay, there is some overhauling to do, but together we can get it done.

Putting Your Inner Critic on Trial: Examining the Evidence

Often the things our inner critic tells us are overstated and hurtful. Have I told you that you don't really suck? The problem is that the things our inner critic says to us often forge our core beliefs, the thoughts by which we view ourselves and the world. And, as you've learned, our thoughts impact our feelings and behaviors. So if your inner critic is in charge of those things, we'd best be sure we know when those thoughts include some truth. Or not!

For this exercise, jot down a common statement from your inner critic. Then fill in the evidence both for and against that statement to allow you to determine whether or not to believe your inner critic. Here's an example:

Inner Critic's Statement:
Nobody likes you.

Evidence for This Statement:
When my coworkers went out to lunch, they didn't invite me.

Evidence against This Statement:
They've invited me before, but they all knew I had a deadline today. One of my coworkers asked me to their party this weekend. Another asked me if I was going to the party and asked if I wanted a ride.

CONTINUED»

Now it's your turn:

Inner Critic's Statement:

Evidence for This Statement:

Evidence against This Statement:

How did you do? Here's another one you can complete to help reinforce what you've learned:

Inner Critic's Statement:

Evidence for This Statement:

Evidence against This Statement:

Turning Your Inner Critic into Your Inner Coach

The original goal of your inner critic wasn't to hurt your feelings or push the mute button on your life. Initially, its mission was to provide helpful, corrective feedback as you learned about the world. It's time to remind it of its purpose.

Imagine having a coach in your head. Someone who assesses your strengths and offers advice on how to tap your best qualities to succeed in life. No, not those bad-mouthing coaches from B-grade sports movies who bellow away so loudly you have to wipe the spittle off your glasses. Think of a coach in your head like the great John Wooden of the UCLA basketball team, who knew the power of orchestrating our own emotions. He relied on values such as character, learning from adversity, and, yes, even love.

Tennessee basketball coach Pat Summitt once said, "Confidence is what happens when you've done the hard work that entitles you to succeed." That's strong advice, and much more helpful than "Give it up, you suck." That's the kind of inner coach we all need.

In this exercise, you will have an opportunity to start turning your inner critic into your inner coach by changing the way you hear and apply your own inner feedback. In the first column, jot down what your inner critic has said or is saying to you. In the second column, think about what a caring coach might say to you instead and jot down that down. You can come back to this exercise each time your inner critic gives you a hard time. An example is provided to help you on your way.

THE VOICE OF YOUR INNER CRITIC	THE VOICE OF YOUR INNER COACH
Example: You really bombed that test. Only a 70%. Wow. Just wow. You suck.	*Example: This is a good place to start. Let's make a plan to improve the score.*

CONTINUED»

THE VOICE OF YOUR INNER CRITIC	THE VOICE OF YOUR INNER COACH
Example: You really bombed that test. Only a 70%. Wow. Just wow. You suck.	*Example: This is a good place to start. Let's make a plan to improve the score.*

Beyond the Book:
Defusing Your Inner Critic

Let's face it. Much of what your inner critic says is just silly. But you've probably found that using logic against your inner critic doesn't always work. So let's talk defusion. No, that's not a scientific formula or a new kind of cuisine. *Defusion* is a term from acceptance and commitment therapy (ACT).

Defusion means to step back and detach from a thought to take away its power. It's just like defusing a bomb. We should carefully assess our thinking instead of getting tangled up in it. We should see our thoughts for what they are—just words. When we get fused with a thought, we can get lost in its power. When it comes to our inner critic, it means we are buying whatever that voice says, no matter how hurtful or disempowering. *Defusion* means unhooking from those unhelpful thoughts.

The goal: Taking a step back, a deep breath, and a scrutinizing look at what the inner critic just said. Let's try to see inner critic's message not as "truth" or "reality." It's just a thought, after all. Once you learn, in this chapter, to defuse some of the unhelpful things your inner critic says, practice these skills in your daily life every time you notice your inner critic in action.

Defusion in Action

Now it's time to try some helpful defusion techniques to quiet your inner critic. You have four to choose from. Use whichever works best or use them in combination.

"I'm Having the Thought That . . ."

Identify the thought that has you hooked. For example, "No one likes me." Saying it like that makes it sound like an absolute truth. And that hooks you even more deeply. Try adding this phrase to the front of your thought: "I notice I'm having the thought that . . ." So, in our example, it would be: "I notice I'm having the thought that no one likes me."

Do you see how now we are taking note of the thought rather than just believing it outright? We're separate from the thought and having a good look at it, rather than getting all caught up in it. That's defusion!

"I Am a Banana!"

Bring to mind a thought that starts with "I am . . ." For example, "I am an idiot." Notice what happens when you think that thought.

Now bring to mind the thought, "I am a banana!" Notice what happens when you think the banana thought. With the first thought ("I am an idiot"), you probably felt some irritation and shame. But with "I'm a banana," you might have been a little happy, maybe even laughed a little. Sure. It's silly. Of course, it is—it's just a thought!

Words can carry varying levels of importance, depending on the weight we let them have. The lesson here is, no matter what, each sentence is just words, ya big ol' banana.

"Thank You, Brain."

When you get bad advice, what do you usually do? You say, "Why, thank you for the suggestion," because you're a polite person. And then you assess the advice. And you just might arrive, in your mind, with "That's the dumbest thing I ever heard." Not that you would say that out loud, of course.

Try the same thing with the advice you get from your inner critic. "Thank you for the advice, but upon further refection, I don't think everyone hates me. And I am a pretty good cook. And I don't suck."

Give it a try. Say "thank you" to your inner critic, and then opt for reality instead.

The SpongeBob System

Someone I dearly love is a big fan of the TV cartoon *SpongeBob SquarePants*. They charge around saying, "I'm ready! I'm ready!" in the goofy voice of that big yellow rectangle of animated positivity. You may have your own favorite character with an equally silly voice. Elmer Fudd? Steve Urkel? Marge Simpson? Scooby Doo? Beavis and/or Butt-Head?

The next time you experience a negative thought, repeat it in the voice of one of those characters, or one of your favorites. "Respect my authoritah! Because you suck!" That's how Eric Cartman from *South Park* might say it. This little trick certainly can strip the power to hurt out of such a thought. It can be a whimsical way to attain a little perspective. And you might get a giggle out of it, too.

Increase Your Self-Regard

You've probably been told that having good self-esteem is a really good thing and that you should work to increase your self-esteem. Self-esteem, however, can be a fair-weather friend. It is your best friend when you're doing well, making friends, winning awards, and getting all kinds of positive attention.

When things aren't going your way? Hey, where did self-esteem go? The problem with self-esteem is that it's usually based on our accomplishments, what we perceive is "good" about us. Only feeling good about ourselves when we are experiencing success leads to perfectionism and can trigger self-loathing when we aren't "perfect."

Instead, let's look at increasing your self-*regard*. This means increasing your consideration for yourself and liking yourself the way you are. This would include noting your positive traits as well as having compassion for yourself when you are you are struggling (we'll talk more about that later).

The challenging part of maintaining positive self-regard is recognizing your accomplishments and positive qualities in tandem with embracing the perfect imperfection of your own humanity.

Increasing our self-regard doesn't just mean telling ourselves we are awesome all the time. But it does mean reducing—or defusing—negative self-talk. We need to:

- Break the habit of comparing ourselves to others.

- Accept our flaws. Everybody's got them.

- Learn to speak up for our wants and needs in effective ways.

- Consistently practice self-care. That means learning and believing that we really do matter.

In the following pages, we will look at increasing self-regard by identifying our accomplishments and positive qualities. We will also be looking at increasing our sense of self-worth by communicating our wants and needs in strategic ways. Also, we will balance self-regard with self-compassion, which is a great way to help ourselves back on to our feet when we make mistakes or encounter a failure.

Self-Regard and Self-Care Log

Sometimes, we forget to notice our small (and maybe not so small) accomplishments and acts of self-care throughout the day. Sometimes, when times are tough, just getting out of bed can be challenging. This week, take a few minutes near the end of each day to write down your accomplishments in the following log. Make sure to give yourself credit even for tiny wins!

Day 1

Today I accomplished: ....

....

Something I did well: ....

....

Something I did to care for myself: ....

....

Day 2

Today I accomplished: ....

....

Something I did well: ....

....

Something I did to care for myself: ....

....

Day 3

Today I accomplished: ....

....

Something I did well: ....

....

Something I did to care for myself: ....

....

Day 4

Today I accomplished: ....

....

Something I did well: ....

....

Something I did to care for myself: ....

....

Day 5

Today I accomplished: ....

....

Something I did well: ....

....

Something I did to care for myself: ....

....

Day 6

Today I accomplished: ....

....

Something I did well: ....

....

Something I did to care for myself: ....

....

Day 7

Today I accomplished: ....

....

Something I did well: ....

....

Something I did to care for myself: ....

....

My Strengths and Qualities

Sometimes life knocks us around so much that we forget how we make the world a better place just by existing. Take some time to create a list of your valuable and worthy qualites in each of the following categories. If you need assistance, ask for help from folks who care about you.

Things I am good at:

How I have helped others:

My most important values:

Challenges I have overcome:

_____
_____
_____
_____
_____

How I have made others happy:

_____
_____
_____
_____
_____

Things that make me unique:

_____
_____
_____
_____
_____

Asking for What You Want

A great way to show that you matter and increase your self-regard is to learn to ask others for what you want and need. Remember, improving your self-regard involves convincing yourself that the things you want and need make sense and are important.

The acronym DEAR MAN is a guide for effectively communicating your wants and needs with others. DEAR represents the script for what you will say. MAN represents what to keep in mind while you say it. The first template has an example filled out for you to illustrate DEAR MAN in action. Then you will have an opportunity to fill it out on your own.

The process of asking for what you want and need takes a little planning. Before you head into a conversation that worries you, write out a DEAR script and jot down a few notes and encouraging statements for MAN.

Here's the example: A friend is repeatedly late when meeting me for lunch—like 20 minutes late. Here is how I would apply the exercise to develop a script for what to say to her and what to keep in mind when I do speak with her.

	SCRIPT
Describe	Describe situation to the other person using facts only. *Example: The last three times we have met for lunch, you have been more than 20 minutes late.*
Express	Express how you feel about the situation. Don't think the other person "should know" how you feel. No accusations! *Example: I really love our lunches. They are the highlight of my day, but when you are late, it hurts my feelings and makes me feel like you don't think my time matters. It also sets my schedule off by 20 minutes.*
Assert	Ask for what you want or say no. Don't think that the other person knows what you want. Others cannot read your mind. *Example: I would really love it if you could be on time for our lunches.*
Reinforce	Explain to the other person what's in it for them. What is the reward for the other person for giving you what you want? *Example: I think it would be better for our relationship if you could be on time. You might have noticed that I was a little reserved during the first part of our last few lunches because I was a little upset.*

	THINGS TO REMEMBER
Mindfully	Don't get distracted by the other person trying to change the subject or making verbal attacks. Just keep repeating your request or saying no. *Example: She might be hurt, so make sure to keep my tone light and my voice gentle. She might also try to make excuses, just remind her that I would like her to be on time. If she gets upset, remind her I am her friend and care about her but still want her to be on time.*
Appear **Confident**	Even if you don't feel confident, fake it. You have a right to ask, even if the other person says no. *Example: I am going to be nervous, so I should do some deep breathing before. I should also make eye contact so I don't seem so nervous.*
Negotiate	Be willing to negotiate and come up with different solutions. *Example: Sometimes she has to take the bus, so I could offer to pick her up on those days. Or we could meet closer to where she lives.*

Okay, now it's your turn!

	SCRIPT
Describe	How would you describe the current situation to the other person using facts only? ....
Express	Express how you feel about the situation. Don't think the other person "should know" how you feel. No accusations! ....

CONTINUED»

Assert	Ask for what you want or say no. Don't think that the other person knows what you want. Others cannot read your mind.
	....
	....
	....
Reinforce	Explain to the other person what's in it for them. What is the reward for the other person for giving you what you want?
	....
	....
	....

	THINGS TO REMEMBER
Mindfully	Don't get distracted by the other person trying to change the subject or making verbal attacks. Just keep repeating your request or saying no.
	....
	....
	....
Appear **Confident**	Even if you don't feel confident, fake it. You have a right to ask, even if the other person says no.
	....
	....
	....
Negotiate	Be willing to negotiate and come up with different solutions.
	....
	....
	....

What Would You Say to a Dear Friend?

Sometimes self-esteem just doesn't cut it, and we need some self-compassion. When you need a dose of self-compassion, follow these steps:

1. Think about a time when a really close friend or a family member struggled with feeling bad about themselves. How would you speak to this person in kind and compassionate ways (the way you would want someone to talk to you)?

2. Now imagine a time when you were feeling bad about yourself or were intensely struggling. What did you say to yourself? What was different? What was your tone like?

3. Take a moment to imagine talking to yourself as you would talk to that dear friend or family member. Imagine yourself using your most encouraging, kindest, gentlest, and most compassionate voice. Imagine believing in yourself the way you believe in them. Imagine treating yourself the way you treat them when they are suffering. What do you think would happen if you treated yourself as a loved one?

Temper Strong Emotions

Maybe it was that double espresso spilling on your brand-new shirt that set you off. Maybe it was watching your colleague getting praise for doing the same tasks you do. Or perhaps it was coming to terms with that roommate who never does the dishes or takes out the garbage. Whatever the trigger, sometimes you may find yourself seething with rage. Or you're consumed with jealousy or resentment. Or you feel a profound sense of shame. In these moments, your heart beats faster. Your face feels hot. Your ears burn. You feel awful.

The truth is, we all feel anger, jealously, and resentment. And we often feel shame because of feeling those emotions. We tend to think that these emotions are bad, but they can have positive aspects. Anger, resentment, and jealously can make us stand up for what's right. And shame can keep us from doing things that might cause us to be rejected by those we care about. But degrees of these emotions can cross over into an unhealthy realm. Then they can hurt our relationships and even our health.

It can be difficult to believe that we can temper strong emotions, but it is possible. We need to take a little emotional break sometimes and step away from the problem that is causing us to feel those emotions so intensely. In other cases, we can practice not reacting to the strong emotion by doing the opposite of what we think we want to do. You'll learn those skills next.

Putting Out the Fire

When we feel emotions such as anger, fear, shame, or jealousy, it can feel like we are on fire with emotion. Sometimes, we need to get some distance from those emotions before we can deal with the situation that triggered them. Grounding can help with that. Some people call grounding "centering" themselves or "finding a safe place."

Whatever it's called, grounding helps you detach from strong emotions. It is, essentially, a way to distract yourself for a while. Although grounding does not solve the problem that spurred the emotions, it does provide a temporary way to gain control over your feelings. It can also prevent things from getting worse. Grounding anchors you, gives you a chance to calm down, and allows you to eventually return and address the problem that launched the emotions in the first place. Grounding can be done anytime, anywhere, and no one has to know what you are doing.

There are three types of grounding:

- ☐ **Mental** (focusing your mind)
- ☐ **Physical** (focusing your senses)
- ☐ **Soothing** (talking to yourself in a very kind way)

After trying each type, you may find that one works better for you. If so, put it in your toolbox. Time to practice!

Mental Grounding

With mental grounding, you ground yourself by focusing your mind on a mental activity and away from what is distressing you. Here are some mental grounding techniques:

1. **Playing "categories" games.** You can name all the colors you can think of or books that begin with the letter "P" or TV shows that take place in New York or every kind of nut you can recall or whatever else you can categorize.

2. **Describe all the steps in an activity.** Think about an activity you have engaged in and then break it down step by step. For example: "Making a peanut butter sandwich." First, I take the twist tie off of the bag of the loaf of bread, then I take out two pieces of bread, then I put the pieces of bread on a plate, etc. And don't forget: I lick the peanut butter off the knife.

3. **Describe an object in great detail.** Look at a nearby object or think of one and describe its color, texture, size, weight, scent, and any other qualities you notice, down to the last detail.

4. **Read backward.** Pick up a book, magazine, or even a pamphlet and read the sentences backward, word by word or letter by letter.

5. **"Draw" an object in your mind.** Think of the object and imagine how you will compose the shape, what colors you'll use, and so on. Then start drawing the object in your mind. Is it a banana? You silly banana!

Physical Grounding

With physical grounding, you ground yourself by focusing your senses on your body instead of on what is distressing you. Here are some physical grounding techniques:

1. **Clench and release your fists.** Notice how the tension dissipates after you grip and release about 10 times.

2. **Touch items around you.** Your clothing, a pencil or pen, or your chair. Notice the temperature, the texture, and how different items feel compared to one another.

3. **Keep a "touchstone" in your pocket.** Pick a small, familiar item (a stone, a pendant, etc.) that you can use to ground yourself when you touch it.

4. **Notice your feet on the ground.** Really "ground" yourself—literally. Feel your feet and your toes in contact with the floor or the earth.

5. **Walk mindfully.** Notice how your body moves and how it feels as each foot hits the pavement. Listen for the sound of your clothing as it moves along with you. Focus. On. Walking.

Soothing Grounding

Soothing grounding involves being intentionally kind to yourself, either through words or actions. Here are some soothing grounding techniques:

1. **Speak kindly to yourself.** Speak to yourself as if you were speaking to a true friend. For example, "This is hard, you'll be okay."

2. **Remind yourself of favorites.** Make a list of your favorite things in categories, such as favorite TV shows, places, pop songs, etc.

3. **Meditate on an inspiring mantra or phrase.** Think of your own or use one of these: "This, too, shall pass," "I'm doing so much better than before," or "I'm ready. I'm ready."

4. **Treat yourself.** Get a massage, take a hot bath, or go for a high-end pedicure.

5. **Remind yourself of a safe place.** Imagine yourself in a place where you feel secure, stable, and soothed, and visualize it for a few moments.

Grounding Tips

☐ **Figure out which grounding method you like most:** Physical, mental, soothing, or some combination. Try a variety of techniques, then have a few choices so you can quickly turn to one of them when needed.

☐ **Practice! Practice! Practice!** Like any other skill, grounding takes practice. So practice as often as possible. Master the skill before the next time you really need it. It will come in handy.

☐ **Start grounding early on in a negative mood cycle.** Practice a grounding technique before the anger, anxiety, or other feeling gets out of control.

Choose three grounding techniques from those described that you think will work best for you, and respond to the following:

I am committed to learning, practicing, and applying the following three grounding strategies:

....

....

....

Practice these skills regularly this week and beyond so that, in times of need, you will know what to do to "put out the fire" and how to do it successfully.

After practicing and applying these grounding techniques, what have you noticed? Do you feel more in control? Do your emotions change? Are you able to calm yourself and focus on something other than the unpleasant emotions and challenging situations? Are you able to return to the situation more clearheaded?

Beyond the Book:
Hacking Your Body Chemistry

When emotions are running super high, the physiological reaction can feel overwhelmingly strong. Fortunately, there are ways to lower the intensity of the emotion to release its grip on your body. Using one of the following tips in a crisis can calm you and ease you into a place where you can then use other coping skills.

A temperature change can induce the "mammalian dive reflex" (think of an animal holding its breath underwater). This reflex can put the parasympathetic nervous system into operation, thereby reducing the physiological arousal that often accompanies intense emotions. (See the resources on page 143 for a video explaining the science behind this.) There are other ways to change your physiology, too.

Before you try any of these techniques, check with your medical provider, especially if you have cardiac problems, suffer from an eating disorder (including anorexia or bulimia), or deal with other medical issues (especially those related to your heart). Cleared for take-off? Try these tricks:

- **Uncommon cold.** To kick off the dive reflex, immerse your face in cold water (but not colder than 50°F) and hold your breath for 30 to 60 seconds. You can get the same effect by filling a zip lock bag with ice cubes or cold water, wrapping it in a damp paper towel, and holding it over your eyes and cheeks. Even a cold washcloth on your face may do the trick. If using the bag or washcloth, hold your breath for 30 to 60 seconds to intensify the effect.

- **Intense exercise.** Engaging in intense cardio/aerobic exercise followed by a cooldown can deescalate intense emotions, like fear or anger, which prime your body to run or attack. Ideally, try to exercise for 20 minutes or more, hitting 70 percent of your maximum heart rate. After the exercise, pay attention as you cool down and note what it feels like. As you cool down from intense exercise, the body is reregulating itself to a calmer state.

- **Hack your heart rate like a toddler.** Calming your body involves slowing your heart rate. You can't make this happen simply by telling it to slow down, but you can trick it to slow down by taking control of your breath. On page 72, you learned how to engage in paced breathing by making your "out breath" last longer than your "in breath." Your heart rate synchronizes with your respiration. When you inhale, your heart beats a little faster, and when you exhale, the pauses between your heartbeats last a little longer.

If you are super wound up emotionally, this may be tough to do. So, here's where the toddler part comes in. Remember blowing great bubbles when you were a kid? Whether you use real bubbles or just imagine them, take in some air and then blow out through the wand, slowly and steadily, through tightly pursed lips. Do this a few times for the same effect as paced breathing.

It doesn't hurt that most of us have positive associations with bubbles. And no one has bubble-related trauma, right? Except maybe SpongeBob. So why not get a bottle of bubbles to keep in your desk drawer? When in doubt, blow the emotion away.

Opposite Action

When you experience an emotion, it is accompanied by an associated "action urge." This is biologically hardwired. There is no morality about it; it's simply a human response. For example:

☐ When we are angry, we have the urge to verbally or physically attack.

☐ When we are sad, we have the urge to withdraw and isolate.

☐ When we are afraid, we have the urge to run from what frightens us.

☐ And when we feel shame, we have the urge to hide away under a rock somewhere.

The problem is that acting on these urges is often not effective in our day-to-day lives. Lashing out? Running away? Not always good strategies for achieving our goals. You may have noticed—and research backs this up—than when we give into those action urges, we reinforce painful emotions. As a result, we often end up feeling even worse.

Acting *opposite* to an emotion's action urge can be helpful in reducing the intensity of strong feelings. It's difficult to do, but it can help you reroute your negative emotions. This can mean getting active when you feel sad or gently avoiding (or maybe even being a tiny bit nice to) those with whom you are angry. It can mean approaching scary situations or even "letting your freak flag fly" when you feel ashamed.

The next time you have an action urge resulting from an intensely emotional state, turn to this page and fill out this worksheet to get some practice embracing the opposite action. Review the examples for a heads-up on how this technique works.

STEPS TO TAKE	EXAMPLE	YOUR ENTRIES
Identify the emotion. What is the situation?	*Anger! Jordan charged stuff we didn't agree on to our credit card when we are trying to save money!*	
Identify the action urge associated with that emotion.	*I just want to scream, really go off! We are never going to be able to buy a house.*	
What is the action that would be opposite of that action urge?	*I really want to confront Jordan, so I think avoiding the situation for a while would be the best plan deal with things more calmly.*	
How do you feel now that you have taken that action?	*I feel calmer. I feel relieved that I have some time to come up with a plan for how to discuss it with Jordan and can maybe avoid a fight. I realize this is not a crisis, and maybe if I approach it well, Jordan will return the items so we can get some money back.*	

Let Go of Negativity

Do you ever find yourself focusing far more on your mistakes than on your achievements? Do you focus on criticisms more than you do on compliments? On bad news more than good news? No, you're not a major downer. You are experiencing the human condition. This tendency to pay attention to negative events and information far more than positive events and information is referred to as the negativity bias. You may have noticed that it can have a strong impact on your behavior, your decisions, and your relationships.

Why do we pay more attention to the negative than the positive? Remember, inside our primitive brains, we are still constantly focused on not being eaten by a saber-toothed tiger or getting trampled by a wooly mammoth. Paying attention to scary things is something that old-school part of our brains thinks is important to survive.

The problem is: Most days, we don't encounter prehistoric animals. In fact, we never do. We no longer need to be on constant high alert just to make it out of our caves alive. Sure, we should avoid modern mammoths such as speeding buses and elevators that make loud grinding noises. But our negativity bias needn't be nearly so omnipresent today as it was for our loincloth-wearing ancestors.

Letting go of this bias toward negativity can be challenging, but it can be a hugely empowering act. It can dramatically enhance your quality of life. The upcoming exercises can help you sharpen your ability to shed the negativity.

Beyond the Book:
Using the Body to Accept and Let Go

Virtually all of us have seen a statue of the Buddha. He looks pretty chill, right? That's partly because of two things: his sweet, soothing facial expression, and his open, upward-facing hands. With this image of the Buddha in mind, try practicing the half-smile and willing hands.

The half-smile is a way of reflecting to yourself that you accept reality by letting go with your body. Emotions are partially controlled by facial expressions. The brain and the facial muscles are closest to each other and communicate very quickly. So change that expression, and you just might change your emotion. In other words, if you can adopt a serene face, you can actually *feel* more serene.

Here's how to half-smile: Relax your face, neck, and shoulder muscles. Then, just slightly tilt up the sides of your lips in a gentle half-smile. It won't be noticeable to anyone but you. It tends to register to others as an expression of neutral interest. It's gotten me through more annoying meetings than I can count. No one has to see you smile. You are not smiling at anyone else. You are smiling at your brain. "Hey, brain, all is well. We're good."

"Willing hands" is a way of demonstrating that you accept reality by letting go with your body. Open your hands, palms up, and fingers relaxed. It is a very open posture and good for embracing the opposite action urge of anger.

Practicing Being Nonjudgmental

We all judge things and people and art and TV shows and, well, a lot of stuff. We may judge things as good or bad, worthwhile or worthless, terrible or wonderful. All that judging can have a strong impact on our emotions. It can feed negative emotions, especially anger, guilt, and shame.

Think about these statements:

- "I was in horrific, absolutely terrible, gut-grinding, soul-killing traffic."

- "I was got stuck in traffic for a while. I was 20 minutes late."

Which created more negative emotion? Which was a more factual and an accurate description of consequences? The first statement was judgmental; the second statement precisely and unemotionally described the situation and the consequences of the situation.

This exercise is intended to help you ease up on your judgments, aiming to reduce your negative emotions. Here are the steps for letting go of judgments:

1. Practice noticing when you are judging something. You may notice far more judgments than you thought!

2. Ask yourself, "Is judging helping or hurting me?"

3. Replace judgments with:

- Statements of fact: Accurate descriptions of what really happened.

- Statements of consequences: How the situation could be harmful or helpful.

- Statements of preference: What you prefer or wish things were like.

4. Practice accepting reality and letting go of judgments, and remember not to judge yourself for judging!

Now, try the following journalling exercise to let go of a judgment of your own. First, identify a judgment about yourself, someone else, or a situation.

....

....

....

....

....

Why do you want to let go of this judgment?

_____

_____

_____

_____

_____

Replace your judgment with facts, consequences, or preferences. For example, replace "He's a jerk" with "He did something I did not like."

_____

_____

_____

_____

How have your emotions changed as you have practiced being nonjudgmental?

_____

_____

_____

_____

_____

Loving-kindness

We just looked at reducing our judgments of ourselves and others, how about sending a little kindness out now? Loving-kindness is the practice of sending warm wishes to ourselves and others. It is intended to increase compassion for self and others. What a great way to let go of negativity! Letting go of negativity can also improve our health and our relationships.
Try this easy meditation to put loving-kindness into practice:

1. Find a comfortable, relaxed posture, and take two or three deep breaths.

2. Allow yourself to sink into the intention of sending loving-kindness toward yourself. It can be difficult, especially if you are hard on yourself. Do your best. Say to yourself, *May I be happy. May I be well. May I be safe. May I be peaceful and at ease.*

3. After directing loving-kindness toward yourself, bring to mind a loved one, and then repeat phrases of loving-kindness toward them: *May you be happy. May you be well. May you be safe. May you be peaceful and at ease.* Allow yourself to feel all of your positive sensations of loving-kindness toward this loved one. This might be a bit easier than sending loving-kindness toward yourself.

4. As you continue the meditation, bring to mind other friends, neighbors, and acquaintances, and direct phrases of loving-kindness toward them: *May you be happy. May you be well. May you be safe. May you be peaceful and at ease.* This might seem a little less natural because these are not people you are close to, but continue on.

5. Now move to a person you feel angry with. Direct loving-kindness toward that person: *May you be happy. May you be well. May you be safe. May you be peaceful and at ease.* This can help you release anger and resentment toward someone you are unhappy with.

6. Now direct loving-kindness to all living beings: *May you be happy. May you be well. May you be safe. May you be peaceful and at ease.*

7. Now, take a few deep breaths. Enjoy the feeling of having sent loving-kindness to yourself and out into the world.

Loving-kindness Meditation Log

Each time you do the loving-kindness meditation, fill out this log to see the impact it has on your level of negativity and negative emotion. An example is offered for guidance.

DAY	LEVEL OF NEGATIVITY BEFORE (0–10)	LEVEL OF NEGATIVITY AFTER (0–10)	NOTES
Example: *January 1, 2022*	Example: 7	Example: 2	*Example: I was so upset at my mom before doing this. Afterward, I was able to let go of some of my anger and let her know I had a problem with her in a more effective way.*

Before You Move On

In this chapter, you've learned about the voice of your inner critic. You've sharpened your ability to defuse thoughts. And you've learned that feeling good about yourself is about far more than just recognizing your achievements. You've also practiced techniques for managing strong emotions that can keep you from making a bad situation worse. You've been exposed to "opposite action," a powerful tool for dealing with intense emotion. And you've explored the impact that judgments can have on emotions and the power of loving-kindness meditation.

Takeaways

- Let's focus on some key takeaways:

- Your inner critic would be better than your inner coach. Remember to examine the evidence for what that voice in your head tells you and focus on what is helpful.

- Having compassion for yourself when things are hard and standing up for yourself when you need to is vital.

- Grounding and hacking your body chemistry (with meditation, exercise, and relaxation techniques) can help you regulate strong emotions.

- Loving-kindness can improve your outlook and your relationships.

Next Steps

- Be open to a half-smile and willing hands.

- Remember to a be a banana or a cartoon character when your inner critic gets too loud and you need to defuse your negative thoughts.

- Count your judgments on an ordinary day to see how much they impact you. You can make tick marks on a piece of paper or move pennies from one pocket to the other. You may be very surprised at how many times a day you judge.

- Talk to yourself as you would talk to someone you actually like, maybe even love. It is a radical concept, but it is awesome for your self-esteem when you do.

- Breathe in. Breathe out. Feeling good? Well, that's the point. Let's keep going.

CHAPTER SIX

Harnessing the Power of Your Emotions

This final chapter is going to bring everything together and help you harness the power of your emotions to live your best life. You'll learn about your motivations, move towards a growth mindset, and get into alignment with your values. You'll become better at analyzing your interpretations of your own and others' behavior. You are also going to become a fantastic listener and your relationships are going to thrive!

Find Your Intrinsic Motivation

Motivation drives us to take action. Admittedly, it can be hard to find sometimes. There are two types of motivation: extrinsic and intrinsic. Extrinsic motivation is about seeking external rewards, including more money, better grades, positive feedback, and promotions.

While extrinsic motivation definitely works in the short term, research tells us extrinsic motivators are not a sustainable source of satisfaction and happiness. This is because of a phenomenon called hedonic adaptation. When you get a big win, like a raise or an award for your achievements, the high wears off pretty quickly. Seeking out win after win to sustain our motivation leads us to a sort of treadmill, a constant seeking of outward motivators. In the end, we get stuck looking for extrinsic gratification over and over again. It gets really tiring and doesn't make any difference to our long-term happiness.

If, on the other hand, our motivation comes from inside—from a true sense of fulfillment, interest, or enjoyment—then we are more likely to sustain a long-lasting sense of satisfaction and motivation. This is called intrinsic motivation. Building intrinsic motivation involves identifying what is important to us, what makes us spark, and what gives us a sense of competence, flow, and even mastery.

119

Improving Intrinsic Motivation by Improving Self-Efficacy

Self-efficacy is our belief in our ability to achieve things. It's when we embrace that belief that we can make things happen. One way to increase your intrinsic motivation is to increase this sense of self-efficacy. This is accomplished by doing things that build your sense of competence, self-confidence, and mastery. So, here is your mission, should you choose to accept it:

1. Do one thing each day that gives you a sense of accomplishment. It should be just difficult enough to be challenging but not difficult enough to beat you down.

2. Gradually increase the difficulty over time so you are continually challenged. If the task was too difficult, make it a smidge easier next time. If it was too easy, tweak the difficulty level to make it more challenging.

Self-Efficacy Log

At the end of each day, take a few minutes to complete this log. Enter the activity you accomplished that day and plan ahead for the next day. It is fine if you do a different activity than the one you planned for. Just make a note each evening to help you track and reflect on your self-efficacy-building progress.

DAY	PLANNED ACTIVITIES TO BUILD SELF-EFFICACY	COMPLETED ACTIVITIES TO BUILD SELF-EFFICACY

Find Intrinsic Motivation by Finding Meaning

Find the "why" that's behind what you want to do. Tapping into a deeper reason and linking your actions to a deeper purpose can often get you to move forward. For example, going to work to earn money is one thing, but going to work to earn money to create a better life for your family links your actions to a deeper purpose.

Answer these questions to find out more about what is important to you. Remember to tie the task to the larger goal and assess how it relates to the meaning you make of it.

How do you want to be remembered?

....

....

....

....

What would you regret not doing in your life?

....

....

....

....

What do you want to give to others?

....

....

....

....

CONTINUED»

What do you want to give to yourself?

How do you want the world to be different?

Beyond the Book:
When Motivation Isn't Enough

Sometimes, *we just don't wanna*. We know what we need to do. We know we want it, but we are struggling to gather the motivation to complete our tasks. Here are some ways to increase your ability to follow through and have the self-discipline to get the job done:

- **Structure your environment.** Whether your goal is to exercise more, write a book (tell me about it!), or be more productive at work, there are ways to set up your environment to remove distractions and make it easier to get things done. Packing your exercise bag the night before makes it easier to head to the gym in the morning. Having an app that blocks your ability to check social media while you are writing can keep silly stuff from stealing your focus.

- **Set up a challenge or a deadline.** Aiming to eat better? Set yourself a 30-day healthy food challenge. Announce it to friends and family. Plan a smoothie party at your house to celebrate! Things like this hold you accountable and reward you at the same time.

- **Find an accountability partner.** Steps can include joining a mastermind group, hiring a trainer, or just making an appointment to meet a friend to go for a walk. Knowing that some-one else's success depends on yours will help keep you accountable.

- **Be nice to yourself.** Change is hard. Even small changes can be celebrated. If you are doing even one little thing now, that's one more than you were doing last week!

Revive Your Flagging Motivation

We can all start strong, but then hit a wall that drains our motivation. Answer these questions to help you rekindle your *get-to-it*.

What do you want to achieve?

Remember your *why*. What is the reason you want to achieve this?

What does your success look like if you achieve this goal?

What does your regret look like if you don't achieve this goal?

CONTINUED»

What motivational quote or song lyrics can remind you that you can achieve this goal?

....

....

What is one small step you can do right now to achieve your goal?

....

....

....

Examine Your Interpretations

Let's say you are eating dinner with your friend. He suddenly stops talking, stops eating, and starts to avoid your gaze. In this moment, you might think, "I wonder what's going on? Is he upset by something I just said?"

That's just one interpretation of what might have happened in that moment, and there might be many possible scenarios. Luckily, your friend is there, and he's a close pal, so it is likely that you'll get an explanation (bug in the salad?).

Many times, however, we are left to guess. And sometimes we get it wrong. Whether we get it wrong or right, certain interpretations can do one heck of a number on our emotions. Making educated guesses about the mental state that underlies overt behavior is called mentalizing. We can work on our mentalization by checking in with ourselves and with others to check the facts rather than making assumptions and interpretations. Improved mentalization reduces misunderstandings and disagreements in relationships.

Here's another example: Let's say you thought you aced that interview. But, in the end, someone else got the job. Your interpretation is "The interviewers thought I was a loser." There are many factors you can't know about. Boss's nephew got the job? Well, yeah. Thinking the interviewers didn't like you doesn't do much for your mood and won't help your confidence going into your next interview.

In this section, we will be working to check our facts for accuracy when we can. And we'll strive to make benign assumptions when we can't tap accurate information. Why fill our head with self-destructive thoughts when we simply don't have the whole picture?

Check the Facts

Often, we react immediately and automatically to a situation or someone else's behavior. The result: an emotional response. To refocus an emotional response, you can ask yourself these questions to check whether that response is justified by the situation. You may find your emotion or its intensity changing as you answer.

What is the emotion I feel that I want to change?

Describe the situation that brought about this emotion using facts only. No judgments!

What are your assumptions and interpretations about the situation? Would someone completely impartial agree with your interpretations?

CONTINUED»

Are you assuming a threat to your life, your way of life, or your livelihood? What is that threat? How likely is it really to occur? What else could happen?

_____

_____

_____

_____

_____

Is this a catastrophe? If it is (when you really think about it, it almost never is), imagine the catastrophe occurring, and you coping well with it. Who could you go to for help?

_____

_____

_____

_____

_____

Beyond the Book:
Do You Catastrophize?

Catastrophizing is a thought process that takes an unpleasant event and blows it up to be worse than it really is. As you've been learning throughout this book, how we think about events shapes our mood. It is vital for us to be able to differentiate between a situation that is merely a hassle and an actual horror. In addition to practicing mindfulness and the defusion techniques you learned in chapter 5, these tips can help you switch off catastrophizing:

- **Recognize that you are catastrophizing.** First, recognize that you are catastrophizing. Is this actually a truly terrible event that you are experiencing, or is it just unpleasant? I worked with a client who regularly described things in her life as "just horrible." Everything: lunch, traffic, her relationship was "just horrible." It took a few sessions to get her to understand that our thoughts help create our reality. Her immediate leap to "horrible" was making her even more miserable.

- **What are the odds?** When you catch yourself predicting terrible outcomes, try playing odd-smaker. Ask yourself, "How likely is a terrible outcome? What are other likely—possibly more positive or neutral—outcomes?" Place your bet on the most likely scenario. I bet it's usually not the terrible one.

- **Best-friend check!** This one helps in all kinds of situations. Run the situation past your best friend. What would they say? Would they agree that your life is falling apart, that you will forever be alone, and that everyone hates you? Okay, then. Listen to your friend.

- **Defuse those "what if"s.** So many catastrophic thoughts start with "What if?" *What if I fail the test? What if I don't get the job? What if Marion dumps me?* The antidote to the *what if*s is looking at *what is*. Stop and do a thoughtful assessment of the facts you actually know.

What Else Could Be True?

A superficial interpretation of an experience can result in the worst-case scenario. This can pull the blinds down on numerous other possibilities, which, in turn, can trigger an unnecessary emotional response. In the following exercise, you will have an opportunity to consider how you would usually interpret and react to a situation versus other interpretations and actions you could consider. The first chart includes an example for guidance.

Situation 1: A friend does not return your text
Here's how things might usually go.

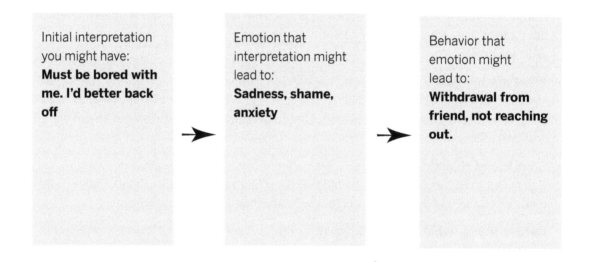

Initial interpretation you might have:
Must be bored with me. I'd better back off

→

Emotion that interpretation might lead to:
Sadness, shame, anxiety

→

Behavior that emotion might lead to:
Withdrawal from friend, not reaching out.

Let's try this a different way! What else could be true?

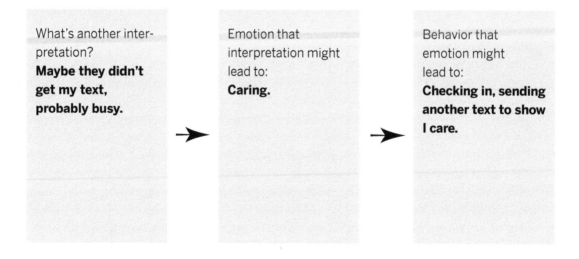

What's another interpretation?
Maybe they didn't get my text, probably busy.

→

Emotion that interpretation might lead to:
Caring.

→

Behavior that emotion might lead to:
Checking in, sending another text to show I care.

Situation 2: You make a mistake at work.

Now it's your turn. Write about how things might usually go if you make a mistake at work.

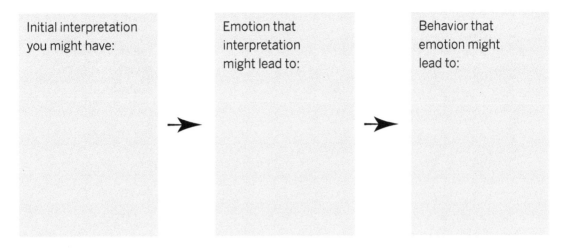

Initial interpretation you might have:

Emotion that interpretation might lead to:

Behavior that emotion might lead to:

Now consider what else might be true. How might that change your response?

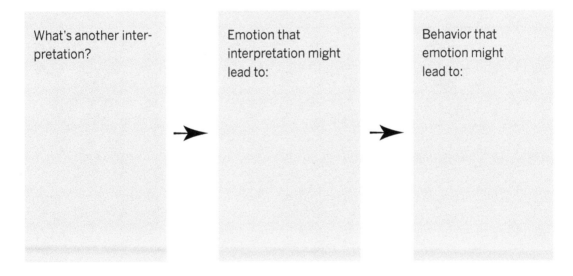

What's another interpretation?

Emotion that interpretation might lead to:

Behavior that emotion might lead to:

CONTINUED»

Situation 3: Another driver pull in front of you abruptly in traffic

Let's try one more example. What would your likely interpretation be if a driver pulls in front of you while driving?

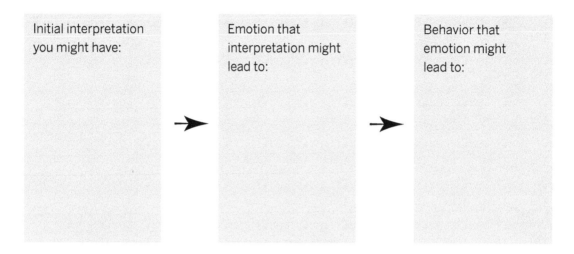

| Initial interpretation you might have: | Emotion that interpretation might lead to: | Behavior that emotion might lead to: |

Now, consider some other options.

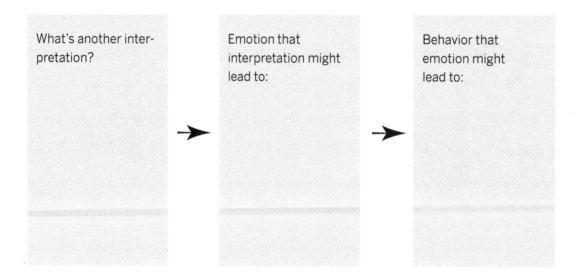

| What's another interpretation? | Emotion that interpretation might lead to: | Behavior that emotion might lead to: |

Build a Growth Mindset

People who believe their talents can be developed through hard work, solid strategies, and helpful feedback from others have what's called a growth mindset. People with a growth mindset tend to achieve more than folks who believe their talents are just innate gifts and maybe are as good as they'll ever get. Yes, you can grow your talents, but you can also grow your maturity, your relationships, your intellect, your bank account, and much more. Growth needn't be random. You can decide how you want to grow and change throughout your life. When you focus on growth and tap the tools you need to attain it, there's a better chance you'll get there.

Values can be essential to achieving a growth mindset. The more we live according to our values, the greater our potential to live a rich and meaningful life. Values inform our goals. For example, if one of your values is being physically fit, you can set several goals to help you live up to that value: make better nutritional choices, increase your exercise intensity or frequency, and participate in a specific fitness activity. If your values revolve around scholarly achievement, that will surely shape your goals, like earning your degree, assessing grad school, and applying collegiate learning to land your ideal job.

Keep in mind that a goal can be completed and crossed off a list; a value cannot. Values are how you want to live right now and pretty much forever. We can achieve goals, but values run deeper. They can define us, which can be a very good thing. Also, know that values can change over time as our lives evolve (aka grow!) and our circumstances change. The discipline to complete marathons may be a value of a young, single person that evolves into making certain that their free time is devoted to their family later in life. Both involve values, crafting personal goals, and embracing the growth it takes to attain those goals.

Let's build your growth mindset by examining your values and goals.

Values List

Take a few deep breaths and access your Wise Mind. (If you need a reminder, see page 39.) Look carefully at the following list of values and circle those that are important to you. These should be values you truly cherish. Don't choose values that sound good or are important to your loved ones, your classmates, or your culture. Circle *your* values. If you don't see what you value on the list, write down your own on the next page.

Acceptance: self, others, life, etc.

Adventure: to explore and be adventurous

Ambition: to achieve through hard work and determination

Assertiveness: to stand up for myself and others

Authenticity: to be genuine, real, true to myself

Belonging: to be part of a group

Compassion: to act in a kind manner toward myself and others in pain

Competition: to be able to compete with others

Connection: to be connected and in relationship with myself and others

Contribution: to give, help, and assist

Cooperation: to collaborate and cooperate with others

Courage: to persist in the face of fear or difficulty

Creativity: to be creative or innovative

Curiosity: to be open minded and interested

Fairness: to be fair to myself and others

Fitness: to look after my physical and mental health

Flexibility: to be adaptable in changing circumstances

Forgiveness: to be forgiving toward myself and others

Friendliness: to be agreeable toward others

Fun: to be fun-loving

Gratitude: to be grateful for what I have

Happiness: to find joy in every day

Honesty: to be truthful and sincere with myself and others

Independence: to choose how I live

Industry: to be hardworking and dedicated

Intimacy: to share myself with others emotionally or physically

Kindness: to be considerate and caring toward myself and others

Love: to show affection to myself and others

Mindfulness: to be here, in the present moment

Persistence: to stay the course, despite difficulties

Respect: to treat myself and others with consideration

Responsibility: to be accountable and responsible for my actions

Safety: to ensure and protect my own safety or that of others

Support: to be there for myself and others

Trust: to be worthy of trust, to be loyal, faithful, and reliable

Which three values are most important to you?

....

....

....

....

....

Now narrow that down to just one so that you can complete the next exercise. Feel free to use the space below to reflect on why that value is especially meaningful to you.

....

....

....

....

....

From a Value to a Goal

Once you have figured out the value you want to work on from the previous exercise, the next step is to decide on specific things you can do to make your life align more with this value. Once you have the goal, you can figure out the action steps needed to achieve the goal and live according to your values. Review the example and then take your turn!

	EXAMPLES	YOUR ENTRIES
Pick a goal	*Connection*	
Three possible goals	*Make new friends.*	
	Spend more time with loved ones.	
	Be more present with my child.	
Pick one goal	*Make new friends.*	
Three action steps that can move you closer to the goal	*Invite coworkers out for coffee or lunch.*	
	Look on the internet for meetups that I might be interested in.	
	Consider volunteering to meet new people.	
Pick one action step and do it!	*Ask a coworker to coffee.*	

Beyond the Book:
How to Make Your Goals SMART

Time after time, we set goals but don't achieve them. Why? Sometimes it's because they are too vague. SMART goals set you up for success. They make goals specific, measurable, achievable, realistic, and timely. The SMART method forces you to arrive at a level of precision that helps you really see and understand the goal—and makes it truly easier to attain. Here are the five elements of a SMART goal:

Specific	The goal should be specific, clear, and well defined.
Measurable	The goal should be measurable. What evidence will confirm the goal has been achieved?
Attainable	Make sure the goal is achievable. Be certain the actions needed are within your control.
Relevant	The goal should align with your values.
Time-based	When is the goal considered complete? How much time should it take?

So, let's say you've been thinking about meditation. Well, that's cool. It's great for emotional regulation—hey, isn't that what this book is about?—and for mental and physical health. Sure, you want to be a "super meditator" type and sit for 45 minutes twice a day. But that's just not going to happen right away. Let's set a SMART goal to get started: "Meditate 5 minutes a day for 30 days."

Okay! Let's check it. Specific? Check. Measurable? Yup. Attainable? It's 5 minutes, dude. Relevant? If one of your values is achieving better mental health, it sure is! Time-based? 5 minutes for 30 days . . . time is all over it. Good goal!

Since you're reading this book to improve your emotional well-being, try creating your own SMART goal around this idea.

Learn to (Really) Listen

Relationships can be rewarding, but they also require nurturing. Sometimes, we are the least able to effectively communicate with the people with whom it matters the most. Earlier in this book, you learned how to ask for what you want and need; now you'll learn about how to be more relationally mindful . . . and really *listen*.

Communication doesn't happen via words alone. It also occurs with facial expression, body language, and tone of voice. We all know the basic skills: Make eye contact, nod your head, and make those listening sounds like *uh-huh* and *hmm*. But do we actually use those basic skills? Obviously, not always. I have to check my phone, right? And there are a million things going on in my head. And then there's that super-fascinating conversation I'm eavesdropping on at the next table. All those distractions are competing for my attention at the same time. This is the opposite of really listening.

Effective listening is absolutely key to maintaining meaningful relationships with family, friends, and colleagues. At its essence, listening is really just taking time to experience what we're hearing in the moment. It's a skill that can be polished. In the upcoming exercises, you'll learn some advanced techniques. Listen up, and you'll ace this skill.

What Is Validation?
How Do You Do It?

Validation is powerful stuff! It enhances communication, soothes emotions, improves relationships, and builds trust and closeness. It is also a way to regulate emotions. Have you ever been really wound up emotionally and talked to someone who totally understood what you were going through? And you found the tension start to flow out of your body and the intensity of your emotion start to reduce? That's the power of validation!

But what is it? Consider it listening to someone with an accepting and open mind, and being able to communicate back that open-minded acceptance and understanding of their emotions and experience. Validation is attained not when you *get it*, but when the other person *gets that you get it*. So how the heck do you do it? Here's how:

1. **Pay attention:** Listen actively, use good eye contact, and use your facial expressions to show that you are not judging.

2. **Reflect:** Paraphrase back what you heard the other person say to clarify your understanding. Let yourself feel some of what the other person is feeling. Let your body posture, voice, and face reflect that. For example: "So you're nervous about the test because you don't think you've studied enough?"

3. **Observe:** Pay attention to body language, facial expressions, and what you already know about the other person. But don't get too attached to your interpretation; make a gentle guess and ask for confirmation that this assessment is accurate. Let it go if you aren't right. For example: Your partner comes home at the end of a long day and slumps upon entering the kitchen, and you say, "Are you tired? If so, we can order in." Your partner may tell you they are not tired and still want to go out for dinner, or they may confirm your observation and appreciate the opportunity to stay in.

4. **Seek to understand:** Look for how the other person's feelings, behaviors, or thinking makes sense in light of their life struggles, their recent challenges, or their current state of mind. Strive to "get it," even if you don't approve of what they are doing or think their facts are right. You do not have to agree with their actions or their facts to empathize with how they feel and understand how they got there. For example: Your friend was recently in a severe car accident. Now she is absolutely terrified when riding as a passenger in the car with you even though you are an excellent driver. Makes sense, considering what she's been through, right? Do you yell at her to chill out? Of course not.

CONTINUED»

5. **Acknowledge the valid:** If their facts are correct and their behaviors would make sense to anyone, validation gets easier! For example: Your partner is irritated with you because you have forgotten yet again to unload the dishwasher. It is time to validate! "I completely understand why you are annoyed with me. I will unload the dishwasher right now and do my best to unload it in a more timely manner in the future." Ooooh, now you are a dream partner. Congratulations! (And keep that promise about unloading the dishes.)

6. **No one-upping or problem-solving!** Avoid such responses as: "Oh, you think that's bad? What about this?" Let the other person have their turn. And don't try to solve their problems; just listen.

Here comes the pop quiz! Read the following statements, and circle all those that would be validating.

I saw how hard you worked for that promotion. That's great that you got it!	You shouldn't feel that way.
That must be so painful.	Just get over it.
He said that? I would be confused, too.	Positive vibes only!
That sucks. I am so sorry you are going through this.	Stop being unreasonable.
I bet you are proud!	You're crazy.

Okay, so that might have been an easy one. The statements on the left were validating. The ones on the right were invalidating. It's a little trickier in real life. See the resources on page 143 for a helpful source.

How to Validate Yourself

Validation from others makes us feel accepted and understood, but we can't always attain it. Being able to validate our own emotional experience is one of the most reliable ways to manage our own emotions. In this exercise, you will practice self-validation.

First, take a few deep breaths and briefly scan your body. Notice any areas of tension or pain. What do you notice about your body?

_____

_____

_____

Take a moment to check in with yourself. What emotion(s) are you feeling in the present moment?

_____

_____

_____

Without judging or criticizing yourself for feeling this way, describe why you feel this way.

_____

_____

_____

Validate yourself for why this makes sense in light of your state of mind, the current struggles you face, or your life history. Again, do not judge or criticize yourself.

_____

_____

_____

CONTINUED»

If the facts fit, validate yourself. Anyone might feel this way in these circumstances, you know. If the facts don't line up, provide yourself with some words of encouragement and think it through anew.

Beyond the Book: How to Practice Mindful Listening

Mindful listening takes practice, but it is totally doable. You can try this anytime you are interacting with another person. Here's how:

1. **Set your intention.** Remind yourself that this is a human being who is important to you and deserves your focus.

2. **Put on your nonjudgmental hat.** Listening without judgments, assumptions, or preconceived notions can help you really hear what the other person has to say.

3. **Devote your full attention.** I know this is easier said than done sometimes, but keep trying.

4. **Your mind will drift.** Congratulate yourself because you noticed you were wandering. Direct yourself back to listening.

5. **Use your body to help you stay in the present moment.** Our bodies are our allies in staying right here, right now. Our minds like to jump all over the place, but our bodies can't be anywhere but where we are. If you find your attention sneaking away, notice a body sensation or two; it will give you immediate access to the present moment.

Before You Move On

In this final chapter, you tapped into your intrinsic motivation and have seen how increasing your sense of self-efficacy can strengthen your motivation. You've looked at how to get your interpretations and assumptions to work *for* you instead of *against* you. You've also seen how shifting those assessments can set off more positive emotions and behaviors. You've learned to set goals that allow you to live your values and move toward a richer, more meaningful life. Finally, you practiced validating yourself and others—and you've gotten through the whole book! That's something to be proud of. You have indeed come a long way.

Takeaways

Let's focus on some key takeaways:

- To increase your intrinsic motivation, find the meaning in the things you do every day.

- The worst-case scenario isn't certain to happen just because you are certain it will. Think about all those other possible outcomes.

- Give yourself a break. Harnessing the power of your emotions takes discipline, planning, and self-love. Do the work, and give yourself credit for it, too.

Next Steps

- Practice validation. It builds trusting and caring relationships with others—and with yourself!

- Determine the values that truly define you. They will help you create your SMART goals.

- Give yourself some major props! You've made it through the book! Now tap those tools and tricks!

- Need a refresher? Come on back to these pages anytime!

Resources

How to Find Help

CliniciansOfColor.org: A therapist directory of clinicians who are people of color; full of clinicians of varied racial and ethnic backgrounds.

PrideCounseling.com: Online counseling for the LGBTQ community.

PsychologyToday.com: The most traditional of therapist directories. You enter your zip code, health insurance, and concerns, and you get a list of therapists.

TherapyDen.com: Provides help for not just the usual depression and anxiety but also focuses on "the problems of today," like white privilege, systemic oppression, etc.

Great Apps

Calm (Calm.com): Provides guided meditations, calming music, and even bedtime stories. Who doesn't love a bedtime story—especially one read by Mary Berry from *The Great British Bake Off*?

Headspace (Headspace.com): Teaches you how to meditate, helps you with sleep, offers playlists to help you focus while you work, and even has workouts.

Insight Timer (InsightTimer.com): A great meditation app that allows you to connect to other meditators around the world.

Trauma

The Body Keeps the Score: Brain, Mind, and Body in the Healing of Trauma by Bessel A. van der Kolk, M.D. (Viking, 2014)

Acceptance and Commitment Therapy (ACT)

Get Out of Your Mind and Into Your Life: The New Acceptance and Commitment Therapy by Steven C. Hayes, PhD, with Spencer Smith (New Harbinger Publications, 2005)

The Happiness Trap: How to Stop Struggling and Start Living by Russ Harris (Trumpeter Books, 2008)

Reclaim Your Life: Acceptance and Commitment Therapy in 7 Weeks by Carissa Gustafson, PsyD (Rockridge Press, 2019)

Cognitive Behavioral Therapy (CBT)

Feeling Great: The Revolutionary New Treatment for Depression and Anxiety by David Burns, MD (PESI Publishing, 2020)

Retrain Your Brain: Cognitive Behavioral Therapy in 7 Weeks: A Workbook for Managing Depression and Anxiety by Seth J. Gillihan, PhD (Althea Press, 2016)

Dialectical Behavior Therapy (DBT)

The Dialectical Behavior Therapy Skills Workbook: Practical DBT Exercises for Learning Mindfulness, Interpersonal Effectiveness, Emotion Regulation, and Distress Tolerance by Mathew McKay, PhD, Jeffrey C. Wood, PsyD, and Jeffrey Brantley, MD (New Harbinger Publications, 2019)

The High-Conflict Couple: A Dialectical Behavior Therapy Guide to Finding Peace, Intimacy, and Validation by Alan E. Fruzzetti, PhD, foreword by Marsha M. Linehan, PhD (New Harbinger Publications, 2006)

Mindfulness

The Miracle of Mindfulness: An Introduction to the Practice of Meditation by Thich Nhat Hanh (Beacon Press, 1975)

Wherever You Go, There You Are: Mindfulness Meditation in Everyday Life by Jon Kabat-Zinn (Hyperion, 2005)

Validation

How to Listen, Hear, and Validate: Break through Invisible Barriers and Transform Your Relationships by Patrick King (PKCS Media, 2021)

Self-Compassion

The Mindful Self-Compassion Workbook: A Proven Way to Accept Yourself, Build Inner Strength, and Thrive by Kristin Neff, PhD, and Christopher Germer, PhD (The Guilford Press, 2018)

The Mindful Path to Self-Compassion: Freeing Yourself from Destructive Thoughts and Emotions by Christopher Germer, PhD (The Guilford Press, 2009)

Self-Compassion: The Proven Power of Being Kind to Yourself by Kristin Neff, PhD (William Morrow, 2011)

Self-Compassion by Dr. Kristin Neff: Self-Compassion.org

Video Mentioned in the Book

"Why Is Being Underwater So Peaceful?": Mammalian Dive Reflex by SciShow (YouTube): YouTube.com/watch?v=tVqw5HnJg-g

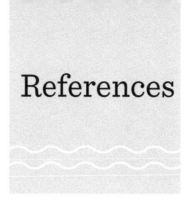

References

Armenta, Christina N., Megan M. Fritz, and Sonja Lyubomirsky. "Functions of Positive Emotions: Gratitude as a Motivator of Self-Improvement and Positive Change." *Emotion Review* 9, no. 3 (July 2017): 183–190. doi.org/10.1177/1754073916669596.

Bandura, Albert. *Self-Efficacy: The Exercise of Control*. New York: W. H. Freeman, 1997.

Bienertova-Vasku, Julie, Peter Lenart, and Martin Scheringer. "Eustress and Distress: Neither Good nor Bad, but Rather the Same?" *BioEssays* 42, no. 7 (July 2020): e1900238. doi.org/10.1002/bies.201900238.

Bradberry, Travis. "Emotional Intelligence—EQ." *Forbes*. January 9, 2014. Forbes.com/sites /travisbradberry/2014/01/09/emotional-intelligence/#3919f8be1ac0.

Broderick, Patricia C. "Mindfulness and Coping with Dysphoric Mood: Contrasts with Rumination and Distraction." *Cognitive Therapy and Research* 29, no. 5 (October 2005): 501–510. doi.org/10.1007/s10608-005-3888-0.

Canetti, Laura, Eytan Bachar, and Elliot M. Berry. "Food and Emotion." *Behavioural Processes* 60, no. 2 (November 2002): 157–164. doi.org/10.1016/s0376-6357(02)00082-7.

Consedine, Nathan S. "Health-Promoting and Health-Damaging Effects of Emotions: The View from Developmental Functionalism." In *Handbook of Emotions*, edited by Michael Lewis, Jeannette M. Haviland-Jones, and Lisa Feldman Barrett, 3rd ed., 676–690. New York: The Guilford Press, 2008.

Côté, Stéphane, Anett Gyurak, and Robert W. Levenson. "The Ability to Regulate Emotion Is Associated with Greater Well-Being, Income, and Socioeconomic Status." *Emotion* 10, no. 6 (December 2010): 923–933. doi.org/10.1037/a0021156.

Hopf, Sarah-Marie. "You Are What You Eat: How Food Affects Your Mood." Dartmouth Undergraduate Journal of Science. February 3, 2011. sites.Dartmouth.edu/dujs/2011/02/03 /you-are-what-you-eat-how-food-affects-your-mood.

Faulk, Kathryn E., Christian T. Gloria, Jessica Duncan Cance, and Mary A. Steinhardt. "Depressive Symptoms among US Military Spouses during Deployment: The Protective Effect of Positive Emotions." *Armed Forces & Society* 38, no. 3 (July 2012): 373–390. doi.org/10.1177/0095327X11428785.

Fischer, Agneta H., and Antony S. R. Manstead. "Social Functions of Emotion." In *Handbook of Emotions*, edited by Michael Lewis, Jeannette M. Haviland-Jones, and Lisa Feldman Barrett, 3rd ed., 456–470. New York: The Guilford Press, 2008.

Fitness, Julie. "Emotions in Relationships." In *APA Handbook of Personality and Social Psychology: Volume 3: Interpersonal Relations,* edited by Mario Mikulincer, Jeffry A. Simpson, and John F. Dovidio, 297–318. Washington, DC: American Psychological Association, 2015.

Fox, John R. E., and Michael J. Power. "Eating Disorders and Multi-Level Models of Emotion: An Integrated Model." *Clinical Psychology & Psychotherapy* 16, no. 4 (July/August 2009): 240–267. doi.org/10.1002/cpp.626.

Fredrickson, Barbara L., and Michael A. Cohn. "Positive Emotions." In *Handbook of Emotions*, edited by Michael Lewis, Jeannette M. Haviland-Jones, and Lisa Feldman Barrett, 3rd ed., 777–796. New York: The Guilford Press, 2008.

Fruzzetti, Alan E. *The High-Conflict Couple: A Dialectical Behavior Therapy Guide to Finding Peace, Intimacy, and Validation.* Oakland, CA: New Harbinger, 2006.

Goleman, Daniel. *Emotional Intelligence: Why It Can Matter More Than IQ.* New York: Bantam Books, 1995.

Gross, James J. "Emotion Regulation." In *Handbook of Emotions*, edited by Michael Lewis, Jeannette M. Haviland-Jones, and Lisa Feldman Barrett, 3rd ed., 428–439. New York: The Guilford Press, 2008.

Gross, James J. "Emotional Regulation: Conceptual and Empirical Foundations." In *Handbook of Emotional Regulation*, edited by James J. Gross, 2nd edition, 3–20. New York: The Guilford Press, 2014.

Gross, James J., ed. *Handbook of Emotional Regulation.* 2nd ed. New York: The Guilford Press, 2014.

Grossman, Paul, Ludger Niemann, Stefan Schmidt, and Harald Walach. "Mindfulness-Based Stress Reduction and Health Benefits: A Meta-Analysis." *Journal of Psychosomatic Research* 57, no. 1 (July 2004): 35–43. doi.org/10.1016/S0022-3999(03)00573-7.

Hayes, Steven C., Kirk D. Strosahl, and Kelly G. Wilson. *Acceptance and Commitment Therapy: The Process and Practice of Mindful Change.* 2nd ed. New York: The Guilford Press, 2012.

Helm, Els van der, and Matthew P. Walker. "Overnight Therapy? The Role of Sleep in Emotional Brain Processing." *Psychological Bulletin* 135, no. 5 (2009): 731–748. doi.org/10.1037/a0016570.

Hill, Christina L. M., and John A. Updegraff. "Mindfulness and Its Relationship to Emotional Regulation." *Emotion* 12, no. 1 (February 2012): 81–90. doi.org/10.1037/a0026355.

Hofmann, Stefan G., Alice T. Sawyer, Ashley A. Witt, and Diana Oh. "The Effect of Mindfulness-Based Therapy on Anxiety and Depression: A Meta-Analytic Review." *Journal of Consulting and Clinical Psychology* 78, no. 2 (April 2010): 169–83. doi.org/10.1037/a0018555.

Hosseinian, Simin, Seyedeh-Monavar Yazdi, Shaghayegh Zahraie, and Ali Fathi-Ashtiani. "Emotional Intelligence and Job Satisfaction." *Journal of Applied Sciences* 8, no. 5 (2008): 903–906. doi.org/10.3923/jas.2008.903.906.

Leahy, Robert L., Dennis Tirch, and Lisa A. Napolitano. *Emotion Regulation in Psychotherapy: A Practitioner's Guide.* New York: The Guilford Press, 2011.

Leary, Mark R., and Dina Gohar. "Self-Awareness and Self-Relevant Thought in the Experience and Regulation of Emotion." In *Handbook of Emotion Regulation*, edited by James J. Gross, 2nd ed. 376–389. New York: The Guilford Press, 2014.

Lee, Hyun Jung. "How Emotional Intelligence Relates to Job Satisfaction and Burnout in Public Service Jobs." *International Review of Administrative Sciences* 84, no. 4 (December 2018): 729–745. doi.org/10.1177/0020852316670489.

Levenson, Robert W., Claudia M. Haase, Lian Bloch, Sarah R. Holley, and Benjamin H. Seider. "Emotional Regulation in Couples." In *Handbook of Emotion Regulation*, edited by James J. Gross, 2nd ed. 267–283. New York: The Guilford Press, 2014.

Lewis, Michael, Jeanette M. Haviland-Jones, and Lisa Feldman Barrett, eds. *Handbook of Emotions*. 3rd ed. New York: The Guilford Press, 2010.

Linehan, Marsha M. *DBT Skills Training Handouts and Worksheets*. 2nd ed. New York: The Guilford Press, 2015.

Macht, Michael. "Characteristics of Eating in Anger, Fear, Sadness and Joy." *Appetite* 33, no. 1 (August 1999): 129–139. doi.org/10.1006/appe.1999.0236.

McCullough, Michael E., Robert A. Emmons, and Jo-Ann Tsang. "The Grateful Disposition: A Conceptual and Empirical Topography." *Journal of Personality and Social Psychology* 82, no. 1 (January 2002): 112–127. doi.org/10.1037/0022-3514.82.1.112.

Mesquita, Batja, Jozefien De Leersnyder, and Dustin Albert. "The Cultural Regulation of Emotions." In *Handbook of Emotion Regulation*, edited by James J. Gross, 2nd ed. 284–301. New York: The Guilford Press, 2014.

Mikulincer, Mario, Jeffry A. Simpons, and John F. Dovidio, eds. *APA Handbook of Personality and Social Psychology: Volume 3: Interpersonal Relations.* Worcester, MA: American Psychological Association, 2015.

Morsella, Ezequiel, John A. Bargh, and Peter M. Gollwitzer, eds. *Oxford Handbook of Human Action*. New York: Oxford University Press, 2009.

Najavits, Lisa M. *Seeking Safety: A Treatment Manual for PTSD and Substance Abuse.* New York: The Guilford Press, 2002.

Neff, Kristin, and Christopher K. Germer. *The Mindful Self-Compassion Workbook: A Proven Way to Accept Yourself, Build Inner Strength, and Thrive.* New York: The Guilford Press, 2018.

Polivy, J. "Psychological Consequences of Food Restriction." *Journal of the American Dietetic Association* 96, no. 6 (June 1996): 589–592. doi.org/10.1016/S0002-8223(96)00161-7.

Rocky Top Sports World. "10 Most Inspirational Quotes from Legendary Basketball Coach Pat Summitt." February 15, 2019. RockyTopSportsWorld.com/blog/inspirational-quotes -coach-pat-summitt.

Scott, Alexander J., Thomas L. Webb, and Georgina Rowse. "Does Improving Sleep Lead to Better Mental Health? A Protocol for a Meta-Analytic Review of Randomised Controlled Trials." *BMJ Open* 7, no. 9 (2017): e016873. doi.org/10.1136/bmjopen-2017-016873.

Scott, M. S., Elizabeth. "The Benefits of Journaling for Stress Management." Verywell Mind. Updated March 27, 2020. VerywellMind.com/the-benefits-of-journaling-for-stress -management-3144611.

Sharma, Neelu, Om Prakash, K. S. Sengar, Suprakash Chaudhury, and Amool R. Singh. "The Relation between Emotional Intelligence and Criminal Behavior: A Study among Convicted Criminals." *Industrial Psychiatry Journal* 24, no. 1 (2015): 54–58. doi.org /10.4103/0972-6748.160934.

Smith, Eliot R., and Diane M. Mackie. "Intergroup Emotions." In *Handbook of Emotions*, edited by Michael Lewis, Jeannette M. Haviland-Jones, and Lisa Feldman Barrett, 3rd ed., 428–439.

Wolgast, Martin, Lars-Gunnar Lundh, and Gardar Viborg. "Cognitive Reappraisal and Accep- tance: An Experimental Comparison of Two Emotion Regulation Strategies." *Behavior Research and Therapy* 49, no. 12 (December 2011): 858–866. doi.org/10.1016/j .brat.2011.09.011.

Wood, Alex M., John Maltby, Raphael Gillett, P. Alex Linley, and Stephen Joseph. "The Role of Gratitude in the Development of Social Support, Stress, and Depression: Two Longitudinal Studies." *Journal of Research in Personality* 42, no. 4 (August 2008): 854–871. doi.org/10.1016/J.JRP.2007.11.003.

Index

Acknowledgments

First and foremost, I would like to acknowledge my brother, Tom Bray, for going above and beyond while I was working on this book. Best of men, best of brothers. Also, my beloved son, Finn, for his patience with me while I spent endless hours at the computer instead with him while he healed from a skateboarding-induced broken wrist. I owe you at least a couple of road trips, little man. Thank you to the team at Village Counseling and Wellness: Darcy Clark, Chelsea Monty, and Vanessa Campos for providing such effective and caring service to our clients. And my deepest gratitude to Dana Dixon and Liz Corpstein for steering the ship and providing outstanding leadership.

About the Author

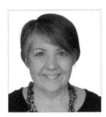 **Suzette Bray, LMFT,** is a licensed marriage and family therapist based in Los Angeles, California. She is the founder and executive director of Village Counseling and Wellness, a program specializing in dialectical behavior therapy (DBT) for adults and teens. Suzette is a sought-after speaker on topics related to emotional health. You can find out more about Suzette at VillageCounselingAndWellness.com.